MW00945205

The Cheer Diet

Female Edition

A 60 day plan designed to help you stunt stronger, tumble harder and look fierce at competitions.

Coach Sahil Mulla

Copyright & Legalities

© 2015 Sahil Mulla, published under Hardcore Training Solutions –
All Rights Reserved. Printed by CreateSpace, an Amazon company.
No part of this book may be republished or resold without written
consent from the author or publisher under any forms of media
(including print, internet, video or audio transcription). Doing so is
a violation against copyright law.

Legal Disclaimer

The information found in this book does not constitute medical
advice and should not be taken as such. Consult your physician
before taking part in any exercise program. The dietary
modifications found in this program are for serious athletes that are
18+ and assume a healthy body. If you are under the age of majority,
have medical considerations that require special nutritional
practices, or have any reservations, please consider reviewing this
book with your nutritionist and physician before starting a diet or
exercise program. Any application of the recommended materials in
this book is at the sole risk of the reader, and at the reader's
discretion. Responsibility of any injuries or other adverse effects
resulting from the application of any of the information provided
within this book is expressly disclaimed. Hardcore Training
Solutions or any of its affiliates **shall not** be responsible for the
actions you take due to the material in this book.

The Cheer Diet
Published January 2015, Hardcore Training Solutions
(www.hardcoretrainingsolutions.com)
ISBN-13: 978-1503209695
ISBN-10: 1503209695

Note: Since this book was designed to be read cover-to-cover, the
table of contents and chapter references are located at the end.

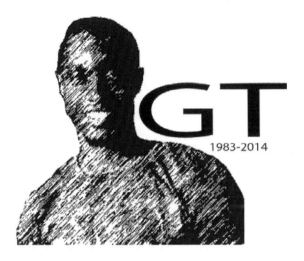

1983-2014

This book is dedicated to the loving memory of Garfield Turner – a fellow cheerleader, friend, coach and one of the most inspiring human beings I've ever met. Although he was taken from us much too soon, he left behind a legacy that can never be forgotten.

I was lucky enough to spend an entire season on the same team as him, winning Nationals, competing at Worlds, and building memories I shall cherish forever. His positive energy was downright contagious – he could walk into any room and uplift everyone's mood within minutes, and his words of encouragement had the remarkable ability to push you past your limitations. It's no wonder then, that Garfield influenced the lives of so many people during his short time with us. And to be honest, if I can have a positive impact on even a fraction of the amount of people that Garfield did, then I'd call this book a success.

So here's to you, my good friend. If by chance you happen to be looking down on us right now, I hope I've done you proud - because the only thing you took more seriously than cheer, was your love of food.

Further Acknowledgements

I wanted to take a second to thank all the amazing people without whom I would've never started this project, let alone finish it:

First, are the loyal readers of my Tumbling Coach blog. It's because of you guys that I actually look forward to checking my email. All the love and support that gets sent doesn't go un-noticed, so thank you and keep those emails coming!

Next, are the amazing coaches (both from the cheer and gymnastics world) that have supported me on this project. Nothing breaks writer's block quite like your peers sending you a message saying "I can't wait for your book... can you release it already?!" Even I need a motivational kick from time to time.

Next up are my amazing friends, who are nothing but positive, encouraging, and always there to help spread the word whenever I write something. For that, I am extremely grateful.

Then there are my athletes, who put up with my perfectionist style of coaching and let me use them as guinea pigs to test new training techniques. I know it can be tough sometimes, but you guys never fail to impress me with how quickly you pick things up (and the competitions we win together). I'm proud of each and every one of you.

Finally, to all the parents that make my job so much easier by encouraging me to push their kids to become the best they can be. There's nothing a coach loves more than hearing a parent say, "Make sure she works hard. And if she doesn't, let us know!"

Introduction

So, why do we need a "Cheer Diet?"

I mean, what could *possibly* be wrong with the hundreds of other diets which are out there right now?

In short, nothing. There are definitely some good, some bad and some great books out there which can help you reach your goals. But if there's one thing I've learned from being a coach (and a high calibre athlete) in multiple sports, it is this: **Specificity Matters.**

This is why if you won't see a bodybuilder do Zumba™ classes while watching his Weight Watchers™ points to help win competitions.

It is also why when I set a National Deadlift Record back in 2012 (402.3 lbs at a body weight of 129 lbs), I was eating much differently than when I was tumbling for a world level team, many years ago. Food is fuel, and the type of fuel I consumed was dictated by my needs and goals.

You wouldn't put low-grade unleaded gasoline in a Ferrari, now would you? Didn't think so.

Similarly, as an Allstar Female Cheerleader you have very demanding expectations such as: tossing your team mates high into the air (which requires strength), keeping a three layer pyramid from falling (which needs focus & stability), doing spectacular tumbling passes (which require power & healthy joints), and being full of energy for two minutes and thirty seconds as large crowds roar, and bright lights shine down upon you (which requires endurance and focus).

Oh yeah, and you want to look absolutely fierce in those uniforms.

After all, the whole point of a performance sport is to show off your best self, is it not?

So cheerleaders not only have to be good at what they do, they have to *look* good doing it. Performance, showmanship, and energy - all of these aspects are part of the overall score sheet in some way shape or from. And therefore, as a cheerleader you need a diet that specifically caters to such demanding needs.

While simply eating your veggies and avoiding fast food is a decent start, it's simply not enough. In fact, that's average. Now if you want to be average that's great, but I assume you're reading this because you want to be exceptional. If that's true, then what I'm about to show you will get you there.

With *The Cheer Diet* you'll reap the following benefits:

- Faster recovery from the most demanding practices (say goodbye to extreme soreness).
- More gas in your tank to get through those never ending "full outs."
- An immune system boost so you don't fall sick every time you catch a flyer with a runny nose.
- A significant drop in body fat.

On top of this you'll also learn how, when and why your body uses certain foods as fuel and when it doesn't. As a teenage athlete, this book will give you a solid understanding of nutrition so you can have the confidence to make proper food choices well into your future.

Now it's possible that you might be thinking, *"Why is all that necessary? Just tell me how I can get abs and not feel absolutely wiped out during practice!"*

Well it's important because you're not only the future of this sport, you are the future of your country. Consider this: In America, according to the National Center For Health & Statistics (NCHS) the obesity rate in the 1960's was around 10-12%. But at this point, it's well over 60%!

Now the United States is often the butt of fat jokes, but I think that's unfair because if you look at the data, countries like Canada, United Kingdom, New Zealand and Australia aren't fat behind...err, I mean *far* behind. In fact, according to the United Nations obesity charts, Mexico recently overtook the USA as the world's fattest nation.

Ay caramba!

So while doctors and other professionals are trying to tackle the problem from the top down - by turning to medication and other complicated methods for adults, I think the *real* solution lies in solving it from the bottom up – by educating young women who have plenty of time to learn how to live a healthy lifestyle and hopefully, pass that knowledge on to their kids someday.

Finally, I want you to know that *The Cheer Diet* will not require you to give up the one thing I know every cheerleader loves... **Nutella!**

No need to squint your eyes, that was no misprint. Everyone knows that a cheerleader without her Nutella, is like a rockstar without his guitar. So leaving out such chocolaty goodness was out of the question.

Just don't expect it to eat it every night... after all, this isn't the *Nutella Diet* =)

Who I Wrote This Book For

I know it seems rather obvious that this book is meant for the typical teenage cheerleader, but I want to take this opportunity to mention a few other groups of people whom I believe will benefit from the information:

Parents: To be honest, without the support of cheer moms and cheer dads, this sport wouldn't be where it's at today. So if you're a parent reading this, I hope you get some good ideas that will help make post-training meal prep a bit easier. I also hope that this book takes the trouble out of explaining the importance of good nutrition to your daughter. Instead of forcing them to eat yet another pile of steamed broccoli, just throw this bright yellow coloured book at them, and let my words take care of the rest.

Coaches: I know your hands are already full with choreographing routines, placing athletes on appropriate teams, planning out competitions, managing a budget, addressing needs of parents, motivating everyone on "off days," and last but not least, playing multiple roles of friend, brother, sister, or even mother/father in the lives of many athletes.

Because of this, I figured I should help take one major burden off your shoulders by making sure you don't have to worry about your athletes suffering from cramps, bloating or puking due to eating the wrong foods at the wrong times. Plus, because their bodies will be fuelled properly, they won't complain or gas out when you say *"one more full out,"* but really meant three more. Or maybe I should say, they'll complain *less*.

And finally, if you're a woman that knows absolutely nothing about Allstar Cheerleading (such as why the girl on the cover isn't equipped with pom-poms) and are looking to follow a healthy eating lifestyle because nothing you've found is actually sustainable, then I promise that the pages that follow will offer you advice that is valuable and insightful.

Who Am I To Make Such Promises?

In the world of cheerleading, most know me through my website (tumblingcoach.com) and my Facebook page (Addicted To Tumbling) where I share drills, tips and awesome examples of tumbling. To this day, the page has received about *half a million* hits.

So if tumbling is my specialty, where does this whole "diet and nutrition thing" come in?

Believe it or not, handling people's fitness & nutrition plans is my main job. I coach tumbling because I love it, so it's like my side gig. But mainly, I provide fitness and nutritional consultation to everyone from powerlifters and mma athletes to regular folks that just want to get in spectacular shape for the summer.

Just like Olympic wrestlers, powerlifters and mma athletes compete in weight categories, which means they must weigh-in before competing. And to this day, I haven't had a single athlete miss weight; they've all been bang-on. So basically, when it comes to weight management and nutrition, you can say that I know a thing or two.

It all comes back to my earlier point that I was trying to make - **specificity**. You see, Allstar Cheerleading has no weight categories, so why would you want to follow a diet created by some guru with the single minded purpose of dropping body weight?

Doesn't make sense does it?

Most "quick result" weight loss diets actually just get rid of the water weight, and favor muscle loss (which is the last thing we want to lose - more on that soon).

The ideal scenario would be to get your body to burn fat, while making sure it stays fuelled for your practices and builds muscle during recovery. But this takes time, patience and careful planning.

So while *The Cheer Diet* isn't designed with the goal of helping you lose weight, don't be surprised if your uniform starts to fit better, you start seeing abs in the mirror, and the random compliments start to flow.

With that said, I wanted to personally thank you for buying a copy, and supporting this passion project of mine. It's been almost a year in the making, and I truly believe that every cheerleader deserves to benefit from the information contained within.

Why?

Because you're all real athletes, in a real sport, that's recognized internationally, and it's about time every one of you had a nutrition and diet plan that helped you become the best you can be.

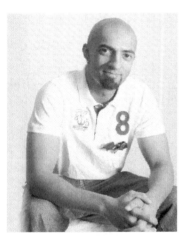

Coach Sahil M.

Certified Level 2 Gymnastics Coach

Former National Champion

High Five Sport Certified

2012 National Deadlift Record Setter

Fitness & Nutrition Consultant

Founder of Addicted To Tumbling

Founder of Hardcore Training Solutions

About The Cover Model

Born and raised in Ontario Canada, Holly began her journey into sports as a rhythmic gymnast at the age of 6. By the time she was 10, she decided it was time to venture into something else.

At the age of 12, armed with the coordination abilities of a baby giraffe, she walked into Futures Gymnastics to try out their cheer program. And boy, was she a mess. Growing faster than a backyard weed, her center of gravity seemed to change almost daily, and this was understandably hard to keep up with. Her lack of conditioning wasn't doing her any favours either.

Trust me, if ever there was a person who wasn't "meant" to tumble because of their body type, it was Holly.

On top of that, at the age of 13 she fell victim to a vegan propaganda video on YouTube, and completely gave up on meat. It doesn't take a genius to realize that removing a primary macronutrient such as protein from one's diet (especially a competitive athlete) is a recipe for disaster, as it's the building block for muscle.

Her metabolism tanked, what little muscle definition she managed to develop completed faded away, and it did nothing to help her performance or confidence. Fortunately at 14 years old, she brought meat back into her diet. But it wasn't until she turned 15 that I stepped in, and schooled her on what equates to proper nutrition along with its importance.

And that's when things changed forever...

Suddenly she was getting tumbling skills every week, her body actually had muscle tone, her energy levels were (and still are) off the wall, her attitude was positive and she basically transformed herself from someone most people would write off as "nothing special," to someone who had all the potential in the world.

I always knew the impact a good nutrition plan could make, but with Holly, even I was thrown back by the sheer speed of her transformation.

To help maximize her potential even further, I got her to start competing in specialty divisions - on top of the team training she was already doing. This basically sky-rocketed her tumbling from level 2 to 5 in less than a year – a feat only overshadowed by the multiple 1st place victories that she came home with.

As if that wasn't enough, she decided to take on a higher level of responsibility by venturing into the world of coaching. Holly took the necessary certification courses, spent more than 200 volunteer hours under myself and other coaches learning everything she could, and now helps out our mini and youth teams.

It's no surprise that they all look up to her as a role model, which is why I chose her to be the cover model for my book. If ever there was an athlete who embodies everything our sport is all about, look no further.

Holly is currently training hard so that she can represent Team Canada at worlds in the next year or two, and I have no doubt in my mind that she'll be able to do just that. Expect to see her in Florida, and when you do, don't forget to say "hi."

In the meantime, if you would like to reach out to Holly, you may send her an email here: **holly@thecheerdiet.com**

You can also follow her on Twitter and Instagram: **@holly_tc**

Finally, she has her own YouTube channel where she talks about eyeliners, cheer makeup tutorials, and... I'm really not sure what else. All I know is that it's super popular (over 30k subscribers) and as a young lady, you'll most likely love it. Go here: http://www.youtube.com/user/TeenBeautyChannel

Chapter 1: Why Everything That You've Been Taught About Nutrition Is Dead Wrong

Let's be real - it's not easy separating the truth from the lies in this day and age, especially when it comes to nutrition. Heck, even Registered Dieticians, Doctors, and Personal Trainers can't seem to agree as to what qualifies as healthy eating, let alone performance eating (which is what's required by serious athletes.)

Some say eating lots of grains and keeping your fat intake low is the best way to go.

Others say it's all about eating low carb, because sugar is the devil and everything else doesn't matter.

Then you have the organic movement to consider because pesticide use is getting a little out of hand these days.

Finally you have the worst possible type of bandwagon ever created in the history of nutrition – veganism. I'll shed light on why it's ridiculous later on but for now, where does that leave *The Cheer Diet?* Well when it comes to the advice in this book, I promise you two things:

1. **It is backed by real research** (All the scientific references are at the very end of the book)
2. **It is tested in the real world, on real clients of mine.** As I stated before, fitness/nutrition coaching is my "bread and butter" job, so I have a vast pool of clients to pull my data from. This includes the young lady on the cover of this book, who really did follow *The Cheer Diet* herself. And as you can see, the results speak for themselves.

So basically what I'm saying is, you're in excellent hands.

Now before you learn the correct way to handle your nutrition, I have to make sure that you aren't attached to any dogmas, myths and misinformation that might lead you to making improper choices.

This means starting with a clean slate so that the new information I'm about to teach you can sink in. After all, a wet sponge cannot absorb anything until it has been wrung dry, can it?

Well, your mind works the same way. If you cram it with too much information and conflicting ideas, it basically stalls. Also known as "analysis paralysis."

So to prevent this from happening, what lies in the pages ahead are my responses to a bunch of commonly held diet myths that have somehow become accepted as fact.

How did these myths come to be? It's hard to say – some spawned into existence due to the media, which bombarded the public with them. Others caught on because they were passed from person to person like a bad game of broken telephone.

However, by relying on real evidence (yay science!) you're about to learn why these myths are about as useful as a flat poof during competition. Then in the later chapters I'll show you exactly what to eat and when to eat it to boost your performance on the mat and experience some of the best training sessions you've ever had in your life.

Myth #1: I need to eat 6 small meals throughout the day to boost my metabolism

I wanted to tackle this myth first, since it is the most annoying of them all.

Why?

Because even though a huge pile of evidence has emerged in the recent years concluding it as false, the "frequent eating" phenomenon simply refuses to die. I guess you can call it the zombie of nutritional myths.

Well guess what? It's time to chop its head off and burn it, once and for all! (that *is* how you kill a zombie, right?)

The Origins

So where did this myth come from and why does it keep circulating around? Well to be blunt, it's because a large group of professionals read the available data incorrectly, then fed it to the masses as truth (this is why communication is so important, ladies!)

See, reading data is one thing, but understanding it is a whole different ball game. This is why I have a tight group of very smart individuals from all over the world with whom I consult with (I'm talking doctors, world-class trainers, big time editors and so on). And by consult, I mean I annoy them with questions, while asking them to dumb down crazy amounts of scientific mumo-jumbo, so that you and I can use the information practically. As the great Chinese proverb reads: *"He who asks questions is a fool for five minutes; he who does not, remains one forever"*

So when it comes to "eating small meals to boost metabolism", let's see what happened, and where things got all messed up.

There is something called TEF (Thermic Effect of Food), which basically means that it takes energy to burn energy. If you want a practical example, think of the gas that your car runs on. It takes oil companies massive amounts of energy and resources (drilling machines, mining equipment, transport trucks etc.) to make it available at a gas station, before your car can burn it as an energy source to help get you from A to B.

Similarly, after you eat some food, your body can't immediately use those calories as energy. It needs to use calories already available to break down and absorb the food you ate, before it can be used to fuel your cheer practice. This whole digestive process raises your metabolism for a few hours.

This little fact is what I believe threw everyone off, because if you ate 3 meals in a day and tracked your TEF on a graph, you would see three "peaks" indicating the increase in metabolic activity. But if you ate 6 meals, you would see six of these peaks (see example below)

TEF for 3 Meals: ----^----^----^----

TEF for 6 Meals: ----^--^--^--^--^--^-----

On the surface, boosting your metabolic activity six times is obviously better than three, so therefore you should eat frequently all the time, right?

Wrong.

Unfortunately your body is smarter than that, and TEF is proportional the amount of food you consume in a 24 hour period. So if you ate 2000 calories in a day, it wouldn't matter if you divided it into 3 meals, 6 meals or even 9 meals. The total energy your body would expend to absorb those 2000 calories **will always remain constant.**

And no, there is no magic pill that can change this biological fact (at least, not yet).

Science To The Rescue

There was a study[8] done, where they took sixteen obese individuals and fed them either 3 meals plus 3 snacks, or just 3 outright meals per day for 8 weeks. The daily number of calories was kept constant in both meal formats to keep it fair and accurate. Here's what they found...

*"...there were no significant differences between the low- and high-MealFrequency groups for adiposity indices, appetite measurements or gut peptides (peptide YY and ghrelin) either before or after the intervention. We conclude that increasing MF (meal frequency) **does not** promote greater body weight loss under the conditions described in the present study."*

And just to put the final nail in the coffin of this myth, here's a direct quote from another very detailed study review[9] on meal frequency:

*"More importantly, studies using whole-body calorimetry and doubly-labelled water to assess total 24 h energy expenditure **find no difference between nibbling and gorging.** Finally, with the exception of a single study, there is no evidence that weight loss on hypo energetic regimens is altered by meal frequency. We conclude that any effects of meal pattern on the regulation of body weight are likely to be mediated through effects on the food intake side of the energy balance equation."*

I'd like you to pay attention to that last sentence. In plain English, the researchers basically found that the only time that food intake had any effect on body weight was when there was an actual change in **quantity**.

So when subjects ate less, they lost weight. I know, what a shocker!

Finally, while I was doing my research on this myth, I accidentally stumbled upon a finding that really blew me away.

In fact, I had to read it twice and scrutinize every little detail to make sure what I was reading wasn't some joke. What exactly did I find?

Well as it turns out, eating frequently is not only useless in helping boost your metabolic rate, but eating less frequently (ideally three meals/day) is *superior* when it comes to controlling your appetite.

The study[12] was pretty thorough and not only compared small meals to big meals, but also compared meals that were protein dominant versus carb dominant. The data from this study is a huge step forward, and has given the field of nutrition some good concrete evidence which we'll be using to our advantage very soon. Here's exactly what they found:

"Whereas higher protein intake increased daily perceived fullness, **frequent eating led to reductions in daily perceived fullness.** *These findings were further supported by the elevated PYY concentrations observed with higher vs. normal protein intake and by the reduced PYY concentrations observed with frequent vs. infrequent eating.*

...these data strengthen the current literature indicating that increased dietary protein leads to increased satiety, **refute the long-standing assumption that increased eating frequency has beneficial effects."**

So it looks like the good 'ol system of breakfast, lunch and dinner that your mom and dad are used to, is not only more convenient, but now it's officially backed by science as the superior method for appetite control.

What more can I say? Sometimes, the new way isn't always the better way.

Let's move on to Myth #2, shall we?

Myth #2: You should always eat 'clean' if you want to lose weight

Tell that to professor Mark Haub[10] who lost 27 pounds in 10 weeks eating nothing but Twinkies, donuts and other "unclean" foods. Or Matt McClellan[11] who lost over 20 lbs while eating nothing but pizza. Or Jared, who managed to lose hundreds of pounds eating nothing but Subway combined with a bit of light walking. I personally have done plenty of diet experiments on myself, and one of them involved eating only fast food every day for a whole month. My results? Net loss of 5lbs.

If you were to look at all the data from every single one of our little eating adventures, nothing would make sense, as it would be all over the place. But there does exist one common denominator that resulted in our success.

Can you guess what it was? (Hint: if you read everything I had to say about Myth #1 then you already know.)

The answer is **quantity**.

We all simply ate less food than our bodies needed, resulting in something called a caloric deficit. It's just that simple.

Now, does this mean I recommend you eat pizza every day for a whole month, or live off candy bars? Of course not. I just wanted to make a point.

We'll talk more about quality soon, when I dig into organic food. But for now, just remember that in the land of nutrition, quantity is king.

This is why when I make custom meal plans for my clients, I allow them a certain amount of their favourite foods (including "junk"). However, when it comes to quantity, there's absolutely zero discussion or bargaining. To date I've worked with hundreds of people, and it hasn't failed me once.

In fact, I can literally make a person fat from something as healthy as a chicken salad. How? By making sure they stay in a caloric surplus (taking in more calories than their body needs). What's more, the scientific evidence on this topic is absolutely rock-solid.

Anyone that says you can eat as much as you want of a certain food and still lose weight is downright lying to you (more on this soon). Either that, or they've figured out a way to defy the laws of thermodynamics... in which case, they should get a Nobel Prize. But I don't see that happening anytime soon.

In the actual 60 day plan, I will show you how to achieve a perfect balance of taking in healthy "clean" foods and the junk stuff like burgers and fries while still looking and feeling great.

Myth #3: A detox is a good way to cleanse the body and lose weight

The unfortunate truth about detox kits and diets that promote detox benefits, is that they don't *actually* do much. That's the best case scenario, actually. The worst case scenario is that certain detox products can be harmful to your health, as certain companies themselves have no idea what they're selling, nor do they have an real evidence of the claims they make.

In fact, *The Voice Of Young Science* decided to find some actual evidence behind the claims of 15 popular detox products – everything from foot pads to pills – by contacting the companies and seeing what proof they had (if any). They combined all 15 of these interactions and released a dossier[15]. I'll spare you the details of all 15 because you can look it up if you wish, but here's basically what they found:

"...We all agreed that detox was being used to sell everything from tea to hair straighteners, and this was implausible. So we decided to dig deeper to find out what the product manufacturers meant by detox – had they some evidence about detox or how our bodies work not available to the rest of us?

We challenged dodgy science claims that had taken hold in public. ***We discovered that companies often used phrases that sounded scientific but actually had little or no scientific meaning.***

In fact, no one we contacted was able to provide any evidence for their claims, or give a comprehensive definition of what they meant by 'detox'. We concluded that 'detox' as used in product marketing is a myth. ***Many of the claims about how the body works were wrong and some were even dangerous.****"*

That last sentence is a little worrying isn't it? Not only are detox products bogus, but companies selling them didn't even have a basic understanding of how the human body functions. Can you imagine a plumber that knew nothing about pipes?

Sounds ridiculous doesn't it? Yeah I thought so too, which is why if someone tries to sell any 'detox' products to you, run the other way. Better yet, tumble away.

The absolute best way to cleanse your body, is to let it cleanse itself by fuelling it properly. Your body doesn't need to go on a detox diet any more than a BMW needs an air conditioning unit – that functionality already comes pre-installed.

You just need to know how to turn it on.

Eating high fibre foods, staying hydrated and supplying your body with the essential micronutrients will allow it to run its own internal detox process – which I might add, is a hullva lot more efficient than any pills or kits you can buy.

If you don't believe me just wait till you get to college. Or observe college kids in general – how is it they can function the morning after a night of hardcore partying?

Because their kidneys, lungs and liver work overtime to remove the alcohol that is floating around in their bloodstream. This is essentially a detox process and without it, college and university classrooms would be empty every Monday morning. So to recap - you don't need to do a detox, a cleanse, or any of that nonsense. Your body can do that on its own. All you have to do is avoid getting in your own way by doing the following three things:

A) Not poison it in the first place
B) Take in quality ingredients
C) Keep your body moving (train hard!)

Sounds easy enough, doesn't it? I thought so.

Myth #4: Organic food is a rip-off and no better than regular food

It's truly a sad moment in time when we have to pay *more* for a pack of strawberries that were grown as nature intended, over ones that were grown with the aid of gene manipulation, and a crap load of pesticides. But that's the world we live in. I'm going to try and paint a convincing picture about organic food, and you're about to learn what's really going on behind the scenes.

First, let's get the whole taste argument out of the way. Every once in a while, you'll notice local TV channels hosting small segments on organic produce by having regular folks taste test it against the stuff growing using modern techniques. What ends up happening is that these regular people come to the conclusion that organic food tastes no better than the alternative, so it must not be worth the price.

Wrong!

See, if I'm going to be altering the genes of a strawberry seed to produce a natural pesticide which kills bugs, I might as well make sure that it tastes sweeter, looks fuller and appears shinier than the original too. In fact, that's exactly what the scientists have done. And this would all be awesome, but unfortunately it comes with two downsides:

1. Lower nutritional value
2. A nice dose of poison currently untested for long term safety in humans.

This is why buying organic produce purely on the basis of taste is ridiculous. It would be like buying a car purely based on its color. The real reason to buy organic is for the higher nutritional content and peace of mind knowing that you won't have any health problems in the future, since we still don't know the long term effects of consuming produce that have been genetically altered.

But unfortunately, simply buying produce that says "organic" doesn't always guarantee you're buying what you think you are. The problem lies in the organic certification of farms. Many companies that have invested billions in genetically modifying foods have started to lose money to the organic movement.

But instead of getting with the times and catering to what we want (true organic food), they're playing sneaky by literally buying their organic certifications for the farms that they own. Here's an excerpt[4] from The National Post about Canada's own organic certification process:

In response to the organic industry's growth, Canada enacted a labelling requirement: Since 2009, products making an organic claim must be certified by an agency accredited by the Canada Food Inspection Agency (CFIA).

***Not included in that process, however, is mandatory laboratory testing of products that could ensure organic-labelled food is actually farmed without pesticides**, leaving the organics industry in the hands of the honour system.*

"It amounts to little more than an extortion racket, one that the greediest of mafias would envy," write Mischa Popoff and Patrick Moore in their report released this month by the Winnipeg-based, free-market-friendly think-tank.

To be fair, the USDA has similar issues. Unfortunately, true organic farming doesn't work that way.

If you have a traditional farm that uses synthetic pesticides, post production additives and other junk, then that stuff leaks into the soil. **The soil is where the true magic happens**. Consider this: If you were to take one teaspoon of true organic soil, you would find that it has *billions* of micro-organisms in it. These organisms help plants uptake nutrition and other goodies and are absolutely essential to their health. In essence, the soil is actually ALIVE.

But what happens when you keep using pesticides and other un-natural modern farming techniques? They leech into the ground, killing the billions of tiny living organisms, turning the soil into a pile of useless dirt.

And what happens if soil is weak? The plants it produces will obviously be weak as well. So how do they get around this problem?

By using even more additives and further manipulating the seed of the plants to produce stronger internal pesticides, of course! And so the cycle goes on and on, until you end up with farms that contain essentially dead soil and crops that produce so much bug killer that it can cause serious harm to humans as well.

This is the reason why an organic vegetable is more nutritious and isn't stuffed with traces of chemicals like its artificially grown cousin.

The real frightening news, is that because humans are at the top of the food chain, we suffer from something called "bio-accumulation." Basically, it's a fancy way of saying that all the bad stuff adds up. So for example, planting genetically modified seed into soil that is tainted with harsh chemicals produce sick plants. Then those sick plants are eaten by animals such as pigs and cows, which also end up getting sick. Then we come along and eat these sick animals, making us even sicker in the process. That's bio-accumulation, and just like drops in a bucket, it all adds up.

The good news is that it can also work the other way round – eating healthy animals that have been fed healthy crops only does our body good.

So how do we find true organic food? Well farmer's markets are great because not only are the prices cheaper (since you're buying direct), but you can ask questions about the farm itself. For example, it could take *years* before a traditional farm can recover the quality of its soil and thus get certified organic again by a proper organization like Demeter International (they're very strict!)

So if you find a farm that got "certified organic" in the last few months, then it's a pretty good indication that there was a buy-out involved. Someone paid someone else money for a fancy sticker so you would think you're getting something organic. Either that or the certification process was a joke.

True organic farms and farmers have been at it for years, and to convert a "modern" farm back to something that produces true organic food takes a minimum of two years if not longer.

To find good farms to buy from, do a little digging, and it'll be well worth your health in the long run. Also, below are a few resources which you can use to find organic products and even have them delivered:

http://www.csacoalition.org/
http://www.localharvest.org/
http://www.ewg.org/
(more links will be added to *The Cheer Diet* resource page:
http://bit.ly/cheerfiles - the password is **tcd2015**)

I hope that sheds some light as to why organic food is not only the better option, but why the cost is warranted. And the price will eventually go down because every time you buy fruits and vegetables, you are voting with your dollars, and so I urge you to vote in favor of organic. Heck, even WalMart is now paying attention to organic food. And we all know what they're good at - rock bottom prices!

Trust me, voting with your dollars is the only way to make giant corporations listen. Tell your parents to buy organic produce when they go grocery shopping. If you have a part time job, offer to pitch in some extra cash to them if they say the price is too high. Individually we each might only have a tiny voice, but together it can be a roar!

And if there's one thing I know cheerleaders can do well, it's have a voice!

Myth #5: You shouldn't skip too many meals, otherwise your body will go into starvation mode

Besides the fact that there's no evidence to back up this claim (more on that in a second), this myth makes me laugh because it makes no logical sense.

If the human body jumped into starvation mode and plummeted its metabolism just because we (god forbid) skipped a meal, then none of us would be alive today.

Why?

Because our species simply wouldn't have evolved to the point it's at today, and we would've died off a long time ago.

You might be wondering, *"what the heck is starvation mode, coach?"*

Well, it's actually a real state that your body can get into where it shuts down the metabolism (so that you burn minimal calories), eats up your muscle tissue as fuel, and favours fat gain over all else, even when you do start eating.

Essentially, it's an extreme survival mechanism evolved from hundreds of thousands of years, designed to keep us alive for as long as possible when we go without food for *very long* periods of time. All in the hopes that the extra time would allow us to find something to survive on, even if it was leaves or a few berries.

Question is, how long does it take for this survival mechanism to kick in?

Well, try and guess. How many hours do you think it takes?

Four? Eight? Twelve?

The correct answer is seventy two!

That's right. One excellent study showed[13] that it takes about three days of pure fasting (as in, only water) before there's even a noticeable drop in your metabolic rate.

But here's something really odd – your metabolic rate and norepinephrine levels actually increase[14] during a short term fast of about 24 hours or so. Just so you know, norepinephrine is a hormone in the brain responsible for helping with concentration.

So let's get this straight - a short term fast not only *boosts* metabolism, but also allows you to achieve higher levels of concentration? Hmm.

How can this be, though?

Well again, think back to times when humans were nothing but club wielding cavemen (and women, of course). The only way we could eat, is if we hunted for it. Now if we went without food for more than 24 hours, this would signal to the body that we are out of food, and that hunting was soon necessary or we will literally starve to death.

And what does hunting require?

That's right, lots of focus and concentration. Basically, it's the brain's way of giving the body a short term turbo boost in order to go kill a wild animal, and bring it back to the cave. And because our biology hasn't changed much in the last hundred thousand years or so, this mechanism has remained intact.

Bottom line: The starvation mode (and consequently storing fat all over you body) isn't something you need to worry about. Not unless you plan on going without food for three days straight, anyway.

Myth #6: I need to do lots of cardio to burn fat and look toned

If this was how our bodies worked, then ultra-marathon runners would look ripped and shredded while gymnasts were weak, thin and frail.

The truth as we clearly know, is the complete opposite. In fact, just look at the cover of this book. How much cardio do you think I have Holly do during her trainings?

Thirty minutes a day? An hour? Two hours?

Nope, pretty much close to zero! She looks the way she does from following a good nutrition plan, along with the hardcore conditioning I put her through when she's at cheer practice.

That's it!

Now, she does enjoy the elliptical and the stationary bike once in a while, but even then, it's part of a High Intensity training circuit which means she isn't on those pieces of equipment for long (a few minutes max.)

The Problem With Long Bouts Of Cardio

If you take someone that sits on the couch all day, and have them start running on the treadmill, they will surely see results. But the mistake is thinking that what worked once, will last forever.

See, traditional cardio by itself isn't terribly effective after an initial period of 4-6 weeks for most people. In fact, if you look at things in the long term, cardio is an easy way to completely waste time while achieving modest results at best, and this has been well documented[16]. Let me quote the conclusion which the researchers came up with while analyzing the effects of cardio:

*"Moderate-intensity aerobic exercise programs of 6-12 months induce a modest reduction in weight and waist circumference in overweight and obese populations. Our results show that **isolated aerobic exercise is not an effective weight loss therapy** in these patients. Isolated aerobic exercise provides modest benefits to blood pressure and lipid levels and may be an effective weight loss therapy in conjunction with diets."*

So how modest are we talking?

Well the average weight loss for the 1847 patients in that meta-analysis was about 5 lbs - and that's in a time frame of half a year to a year, which works out to a piss-poor 0.83 to 0.42 lbs loss per month!

That's hardly anything to brag on Tweet about. I mean, do you want "modest" results? Is that why you bought this book? I didn't think so.

"Ok coach, I get it, cardio isn't a great fat burning tool, but I want to improve my overall heart health and increase my performance for cheerleading!"

I'm glad you brought that up. I want to tell you the story about James Fuller Fixx - the author of the 1977 best-selling book, *The Complete Book of Running*. He is often credited with helping start America's fascination with cardio and popularizing the sport of running by demonstrating the health benefits of regular jogging.

But there was only one problem; On July 20, 1984, Fixx died at the ripe old age of 52 due to a fulminant **heart attack**, after his daily run in Vermont. The autopsy revealed that his coronary arteries were nearly all clogged up[17].

That's hardly a convincing case for a man who said running helps you live longer. Granted, he did have some bad habits when he was in his late twenties such as smoking, but you would think after a few decades of living a healthy lifestyle, he would at least make it to 70.

It's also natural to think of Mr. Fixx as an isolated case, but unfortunately, science has shown that running constantly for long periods of time is actually damaging to your heart!

There was a study done where they took a group of men who were part of a marathon club (age ranging from mid 20's to high 60's), and performed an MRI of their heart. They then compared the image to a control group of men that didn't do endurance exercise.

What they found was rather interesting: **Half** of these older men who did marathon training most of their lives had signs of fibrosis (scarring) within the heart muscle[18] ...and if fibrosis ever becomes severe, it can lead to odd heart function and eventually complete failure.

This likely explains why Alberto Salazer, who was one of the fastest marathon runners in the world (won the NYC marathon in 1981 and almost broke the world record) nearly died from a heart attack when he was 49 years old – not really an "old" age for a man who should be "in shape".

It's also the reason why famous Greek messenger Pheidippides, who ran something like **300km in two days** in 490 BC to deliver a message during a war, ended up dropping dead after he reached his destination.

Reality Alert!

Before you go burn your running shoes and give up everything but light walking and yoga, we need to get realistic for a second. I didn't lay down all this evidence to scare you, but to show you that there is a better way, and that cardio training for hours and hours isn't all its hyped up to be.

Does this mean that if you go out for a 10 minute jog with a friend that your heart will fail? Of course not; that's like saying if you have a can of pop, you'll instantly get diabetes.

My goal is to make you a better cheerleader, and there is not a routine that I have seen in my life, where all you do is run around at a snail's pace for two minutes and thirty seconds.

Cheer is an high-intensity interval sport. There are periods of high physical output, and periods where the body isn't doing much (holding positions, waiting in nugget etc.)

So doesn't it make sense that we should train in high intensity intervals?

Well, duh.

Jogging for an hour at 50% of your capacity will only train you to be slow. I'll talk more on effective training methods later on in the book, but for now, if doing lots and lots of cardio was something you were doing in the past, then you should rejoice, as I just gave you back a few hours of your life.

You can now spend this time on more productive things like homework... hah!

Myth #7: If I eat fatty foods, I'll get fat

The funny thing about nutrition is that just because something sounds "right", doesn't necessarily make it so. If simply consuming calories from fat made you fat, then consuming most of your calories from sugar should make you sweeter than a honey bun. But we all know that isn't true.

In chapter 3 you'll learn more about the different types of edible fats and how your body uses it as fuel, but for now here are a few reasons why it's important for you to not be afraid to consume healthy amounts of fat (especially as an athlete):

- Keeps hormone levels balanced
- Aids recovery
- Provides fuel for demanding workouts
- Helps you blunt the feeling of hunger

Some good sources of fat include:
- Coconut oil
- Omega 3 fish oil
- Organic butter
- Saturated Fat from meat
- Olive Oil

"Hold on just a minute coach..." you might be saying. *"Did you just say that saturated fat is good for you? I heard it can clog your arteries!"*

First, let me just say that anything in excessive amounts is bad for you, even water! But in normal amounts, yes, I'm saying that everything you've heard about saturated fat is downright wrong. It is actually *necessary* for you to consume.

Think about this for a second, if saturated fat was so bad, why do your own cells have the ability produce it in the first place?

Doesn't make sense does it?

Second of all, a meta-analysis[5] that looked at a total of *twenty one studies* on this subject (that's a lot) found that saturated fat has nothing to do with increasing your risk of cardiovascular disease. Here's a quote:

"A meta-analysis of prospective epidemiologic studies showed that there is no significant evidence for concluding that dietary saturated fat is associated with an increased risk of CHD or CVD. More data are needed to elucidate whether CVD risks are likely to be influenced by the specific nutrients used to replace saturated fat."

Note: when they meant CVD, they were referring to "cardiovascular disease." So not only does saturated fat not cause harm, it actually has another trick up its sleeve that most people didn't even know about – **it can actually help lower your risk of heart disease.**

How?

By raising your cholesterol levels. I know, sounds weird right? That's because most of the population thinks that cholesterol is something bad, and that it should be avoided. Now as I said before, anything in excess can cause harm, but when it comes to cholesterol, it is a molecule that is absolutely essential to our bodies. In fact, without it we wouldn't be able to live!

But you have to remember there are two types of cholesterol, LDL (the bad kind) and HDL (the good kind). Why is LDL bad? Because it collects in the walls of blood vessels and can cause blockages. Basically, it would be like having the plumbing system of your house all clogged up.

And if this clog gets bad, you could end up with a blood clot which can result in a heart attack. Not fun.

On the contrary, how is HDL good? Because it transports the bad cholesterol (LDL) *away* from the arteries and towards the liver, where it can be reused or just plain thrown out. So a rise in HDL cholesterol is something you want, not something you want to avoid.

Fortunately for us, saturated fat does exactly that – **it boosts the HDL levels in your blood**.[7,8]

Sounds to me like saturated fat is pretty awesome... and it's delicious too!

Myth #8: Gluten is bad for you and should always be avoided

I still don't understand the recent rise of gluten-free foods: they taste worse, and cost more; much confuse.

Now, if you have gluten-free products in your home, or just enjoy them in general because you think they're healthier, let me ask you a quick question:

Do you have celiac disease?

If so, then avoiding gluten is *absolutely* a good idea, just as avoiding peanuts is a pretty good idea if you have a nut allergy. But the only way to know if you have celiac disease, is to talk to your doctor, as he or she will test you for it.

However, if you don't have celiac disease, then there's no reason for you to actively avoid and pay more for gluten-free foods. In fact, it could end up being harmful as most gluten-free foods lack essential vitamins, minerals and fibre compared to their normal counterparts[1]. And as an athlete, having a diet lacking in minerals, vitamins and fibre is the last thing you need.

Here's another fun fact: Only about 1% of North Americans have celiac disease, [1] yet 18% of Americans are now buying gluten-free foods[2], and the entire industry has grown by 28% from 2004 to 2011. You don't have to be a genius to realize that the numbers just don't add up, and that people are being duped into spending extra money for no apparent reason.

Now besides celiac disease, some may say that they need to avoid gluten because they have NCGS (non-celiac gluten sensitivity). Basically, this means that they experience similar symptoms of someone who has celiac disease, without *actually* having the disease. I know, I had to scratch my head at that one as well.

Turns out, the head scratching was warranted as there was a study carried out recently to see if NCGS is a valid condition[3]. Here's how it all went down:

They took 37 people and put them on three very strict diets (high gluten, low gluten, and no gluten). Each of these diets had many random variables removed such as lactose (in case any of the subjects had an intolerance to it), preservatives, and carbohydrates that would be poorly absorbed. On top of that, the researchers collected nine days worth of poop from each of the subjects, just to make ensure completeness and accuracy. Hey, if you're going to control and measure what goes in, you need to do the same for what comes out. Science can be a messy business sometimes.

So what did they find after analyzing all the data and looking at all that poop?

Did the high gluten diets cause any problems?

Well yes, it did. But here's the funny thing – so did the other diets! In fact, **all diets caused some pain, bloating and gas to a similar degree.** Even after analyzing all the poop, the researchers found nothing out of the ordinary (I think the appropriate term here is, *"shit just got real!"*)

Here's a direct quote from the main researcher: *"we found no evidence of specific or dose-dependent effects of gluten in patients with NCGS"*

So how could this be? Well after careful analysis, they found out that people have a "nocebo" effect to gluten. If you've heard about the "placebo" effect, then this is just the opposite. Either way, it basically means **it's all in their heads.**

For example, if I convince a person that blue M&M's cause stomach problems in 95% of the population, and keep bombarding them with this "fact," then it's very likely that if this person happens to eat a blue piece of candy at some point in the future, they'll feel something funny going on in their tummy – that's the nocebo effect in a nutshell.

It's the same with gluten - the media has portrayed it as "bad" and so whenever people eat foods that aren't listed as "gluten free" on the box, they start to feel like they're having stomach problems and freak out.

Now if you've been a gluten-free advocate for a while, I understand if all this is a bit hard to swallow, but I assure you that just like Shakira's hips - science don't lie. From the current data available, I firmly believe that gluten-free foods aren't all they're hyped up to be. Instead of wasting your cash on them, why not save your money for a fabulous new bow instead?

Myth #9: Buying "calorie free" drinks or foods is a smart and safe way to avoid sugar and save calories

Technically speaking yes, you will save on calories by buying sugar free drinks or beverages, and as you'll soon discover, the total amount of calories you take in can have a direct result on your body's ability to maintain or lose weight (amongst other factors).

But when it comes to long term health and wellbeing, the trade-off you get by consuming the sugar free alternatives is not worth it in my opinion. Let's take a look at Aspartame for example – the most commonly used ingredient in "sugar free" drinks and candy.

It has about ten thousand complaints filed against it to the FDA. It's been known to cause muscle spasms, blindness, weight gain, loss of taste along with 70 other adverse effects (again, all documented by the FDA.) When fed to rats, it resulted in tumours and brain damage.

Yet somehow, FDA gave it the GRAS status (Generally Recognized As Safe) and now, it's allowed in over 5000 products across North America.

How's that possible? Well, let's dig a little further as to how this compound ended up in our foods - it's quite a thriller of a tale, fit for a Hollywood movie script.

(Note: if you couldn't care less about the history of aspartame or how it works, just move on to the next myth. The bottom line is that I believe you should avoid it as much as possible.)

When aspartame was first discovered and tested, it was *not* allowed to be marketed or sold. The head of the FDA at the time (Jere E. Goyan) looked over the studies and saw the highly increased rate of cancer in rats that ingested aspartame.

He disallowed the use of aspartame and was then mysteriously fired shortly after. And those studies Goyan looked at are now nowhere to be found. Isn't that shockingly convenient?

Instead, the original studies were replaced by ones that seemed like they were performed by a bunch of kids on a candy high. This point was proven years down the road (after Aspartame got approved) when some investigators found that the rats used during the studies had tumours which were *intentionally cut out* - and then documented as if they had none in the first place[19].

It doesn't get any shadier than that... or does it?

Well, it does. See, when rats would die of brain tumours or other issues that came up in their organs, these scientists (paid by aspartame lobbyists) wouldn't autopsy their body for years, letting the tumour tissue naturally deteriorate. Then when they felt like it, the researchers would cut them open and document the results of the study and be like, *"See guys? Hardly any tumours at all! It's totally safe"*

It also doesn't help that Searle (the company that patented aspartame) paid money to senators that were involved with keeping the compound on the market, along with huge donations (actual amount unknown) to the *American Diabetes Association* and *The Multiple Sclerosis Foundation.*

As you can imagine, these are names that people trust, so when you see the Diabetes Association website tout the horn of aspartame, it results in a huge sales boost, and people end up believing *their* word over actual evidence. And who can blame them?

Fortunately, you now know the truth about aspartame's real safety. Let's take a look at why it wrecks such destruction in your body.

First, you should know that just like smoking cigarettes, the effects of aspartame aren't always instant. It could take months or years before you suffer any consequences.

Aspartame is made up of three compounds: aspartic acid, phenylalanine and methanol.

Now your brain already contains something called aspartate – which acts as a neurotransmitter (helps brain cells talk to each other). However, when you take in aspartic acid from aspartame, it increases the levels of aspartate you already had in you. And when you have too much of that neurotransmitter, it is now classified as an excitotoxin.

Basically, it "excites" the brain cells to death, which is definitely not a good thing. So it should be of no surprise then, that those 10,000+ complaints filed to the FDA mostly consisted of neurological issues; everything from severe headaches to difficulty thinking, seizures, memory loss etc.

Who knew that continually killing brain cells would cause such issues? I for one am *totally* shocked (not). If you keep up this brain-cell killing frenzy long enough, it can lead to things like Alzheimer's disease, Epilepsy, Dementia and whole bunch of other mental issues that'll turn you into a prune.

The next part of aspartame is methanol, which when ingested is converted into formaldehyde in both humans and rats (don't forget this fact). Now, if you've never heard of formaldehyde then it's about time you did – it's a known **carcinogen** (known to cause cancer) and below are a few of the other nasty things it is known to cause:

- Permanent blindness by damaging the optic nerve
- Chronic Poisoning
- Chronic toxicity
- Skin Rashes

Now here's where things get a little interesting: methanol (the precursor to formaldehyde) is naturally found in wine and fruit juices. I know what you're thinking...

"Mother nature, how could you!?"

But isn't it interesting how we don't experience those (oh so desirable) symptoms from actually drinking natural fruit juices or in your parent's cases, wine?

Well there's app for that... er, I mean a reason for that.

You see, the methanol in wine and fruit juice is attached to something call pectin. What pectin does, is it blocks the conversion of methanol to formaldehyde in the first place, which means it passes right through your body and you just pee it out.

You can think of pectin like a bouncer at a club, grabbing methanol by the arm and kindly escorting it out of your system. It seems like Mother Nature knows what she is doing after all. On top of that, fruits and wines also contain natural amounts of ethanol (that's the magical ingredient that gets adults all drunk, and you can't have it till you're 21... or 19 in Canada.)

But why is this important to know? Because ethanol counter acts with methanol and essentially cancels it out. In fact, one of the treatments for methanol poisoning is to IV the patient with ethanol till their blood alcohol level shoots up.

Or in layman's terms, to save the patient's life, the solution is to get them very drunk. Now there's a visit to the hospital I'm sure some adults wouldn't mind. So ethanol is the reason why you can consume an entire fruit basket, and not worry about going simultaneously blind and dumb.

But The Million Dollar Question Is: does aspartame contain any of the protective substances that stops the formaldehyde conversion? Unfortunately not.

And want to know the worst part about formaldehyde? Your body doesn't know how to get rid of it, so it just stores it. You know, just in case you needed some poison for a rainy day in the near future.

The Counter Argument To Aspartame's Safety

I hope I've made a convincing enough case as to why you should avoid aspartame. But in the interest of a balanced perspective, I will say that there is also counter evidence to what I wrote in the previous pages, which shows that aspartame is safe.

There are also a few nutritionists and doctors (whom I personally learnt from, and look up to) that currently hold the opinion that aspartame is perfectly ok to consume in reasonable quantities - such as those you'll find in diet soda[20].

So if these are men I look up to, why does my opinion still differ? Because even if I'm completely wrong (I doubt it), my stance on aspartame results in a net positive by default. Here's what I mean:

If long term studies do end up with undeniable data which showcases that aspartame is terrible for human consumption, you and I will be better off since we didn't consume it anyway. But those that did? They're screwed.

On the other hand, if long term studies end up with undeniable data which prove that aspartame is safe beyond any doubt, then again, you and I are no worse off because we avoided it. So my real question is, why take the chance?

Why gamble when you don't have to?

Your body is not only designed for metabolizing sugar, it's damn good at it. Better yet, I'll show the best time to consume it, so those extra calories will be available as extra fuel for your practices instead of extra fat on your belly.

Makes perfect sense to me.

Myth #10: My body doesn't count calories, so I don't need to either.

On the surface level this statement is correct (sort of). Yes, your body has no clue what a calorie is, in the same way that it doesn't know how tall an inch is. This is obviously because "inches" and "calories" are a unit of measurement created by humans in order to have an easier time understanding nature.

So what exactly is a calorie? It's the amount of energy required to heat up one kilogram (~2.2 lbs) of water by one degree Celsius (3.1 Fahrenheit). Basically, each calorie has a certain amount of *potential energy* stored inside which can be used at some point in the future. It's sort of like a droplet of oil - which has the potential to power a car's engine, or turn into plastic, or be useful in many other ways.

So while the body doesn't count calories, it *does* know how much potential energy is coming in and being used. For example, when you eat a juicy burger, your body has three choices about what to do with all the potential energy you've taken in. These three choices are:

1. To burn it off (fuel for workouts or metabolism)
2. To store it (as fat)
3. To completely get rid of it (poop it out)

In reality all 3 of those options play a role (since not all of the burger can be used as fuel, or be pooped out etc.) But besides those three there are no other possible options because as the law of thermodynamic states, **"energy cannot be created, nor destroyed, regardless of what form it comes in."**

So what about all those diets and TV commercials that promote a way to lose weight without having to count calories? Are they all wrong?

There certainly are diets that help people lose weight without counting calories, but that's only because they are shifting your focus away from counting numbers to following certain rules such as: avoid sugar, alcohol, processed meats etc.

But if you peel back the curtain, you will find that what they end up achieving is a sneaky way of helping your body use up more energy than you can put in.

Let's take the Paleo diet for example. In the Paelo diet, you're only supposed to eat foods that were available to our caveman ancestors hundreds of thousands of years ago. This means your choices are limited to the following:

- Meat
- Eggs
- Fruits
- Vegetables
- Nuts/Seeds
- Water/Tea
- Certain Spices (even that is stretching it)

No wonder people report weight loss success stories when following the Paleo diet – they're cutting out like 90% of the foods available at most modern supermarkets such as:

- Milk
- Cheese
- Root Vegetables
- Soda
- Grains
- Desserts
- Juices
- And much, much more

Now I don't want to knock the Paleo diet too much, as it's certainly a much better nutritional strategy than the crap most people decide to eat, but the point here is that it's almost impossible to NOT be in a caloric deficit when you're following it.

This is why I urge you to be cautious when anyone comes up and starts promoting a supplement or diet plan where they say, *"don't worry about exercise, you can eat all you want, and still lose weight!"*

It sounds almost as ridiculous as saying, *"don't worry if you don't have a job, because with my system you can spend all the money you want, and still become rich!"*

Now I don't know about you, but if a person is spending more money than they are earning, they will eventually become poor. They might *feel* rich for a few weeks because of the fancy new stuff they have, but the net bank balance will never lie.

Your body works in a similar fashion; you can try all the trickery you want, but just like a bank, it keeps a strict record of your balance, and it cannot be so easily fooled.

"Wait coach, does this mean I'll have to count calories on The Cheer Diet?!"

Not really. While I wanted to make a point that the amount of calories *do matter*, I also know that you have more important things to worry about. Plus, the whole point of *The Cheer Diet* is to help you perform your best, look your best, and make it easy.

There's no way I can help you accomplish such a goal while you're sitting there and number crunching all day long. Instead, there are very specific phases which have their own rules I've set out. These rules will take care of everything, so you can train stress free while having the confidence to know that your body will perform at its very best.

Chapter 2: How To Fool-Proof Your Success

Are You Committed?

Congrats on making it past chapter 1. I know it wasn't easy, but hopefully I provided enough evidence to help you separate the truth from all of the dreadful lies that passes as nutrition advice these days. Mentally, what we've done is cleared your head – just like wringing out dirty water from a sponge. You should feel light and liberated, because now you're in the perfect position to soak up the *real* truth about why, how and what you should eat in order to increase performance.

Before we get into the nuts and bolts of the diet, the first thing I'd like you to do is get *absolutely committed* to applying what you're about to learn. This is the exact same advice I give to my athletes when they're learning a new tumbling skill. For example, have you ever seen someone do a careless back tuck? *(That's the technical name for a backflip for the non-cheer folks).*

What is usually the result? Well 99% of the time, their carelessness will end up as a fail video on YouTube. Or they'll eat mat and hurt themselves. Or both. Every experienced tumbler has realized the following fact at some point or another: you can know all the phases of a skill, and practice every drill under the sun, but when the time comes to perform it, you'll end up in a world of hurt if you're not absolutely committed. Fortunately, the world of nutrition is far more forgiving than tumbling, but the consequences of not committing are still pretty distressing: you'll waste your time, not see results, and get emotionally frustrated. So we want to avoid this as food is delicious, and I *do* want you to enjoy it.

So the first step in fool-proofing your success is to get absolutely committed, like 100%! Fortunately, committing isn't complicated - it's usually just a decision you can make immediately. Like, right this second. Once you've decided to commit, half the battle is already won, and we can move on to understanding the incredible power of habits (both the good, and the bad).

We're Robots and Don't Even Know It

Have you ever caught someone biting their nails? Or maybe you're a nail biter yourself and at times, find a finger in your mouth only to wonder how the heck it got there in the first place.

This is obviously not a conscious choice – we all know biting your nails is gross due to the bacteria that your fingers come in contact with as you go about your day.

So why does it keep happening?

Simple, it's *a habit.*

Habits are *very* powerful. So powerful, that they can override most of your conscious decisions in life if you aren't paying attention. In fact, more than half of your daily actions are dictated by habit. This might make humans sound like pre-programmed robots, but that's actually not too far from the truth.

Fortunately, bad habits can be replaced with good habits. There are only two hurdles that stand in our way: first, our brain doesn't *understand* the difference between a good habit from a bad one, it just picks up on actions you do over and over again, then turns it into a pattern. Due to this non-judgemental nature of our brain, we have to be careful not to program ourselves with habits we don't want.

The second hurdle we face, is that re-programming a habit takes daily conscious effort (willpower), which can be tricky if you don't know the exact steps.

In fact, it takes an average of 66 days of conscious effort to turn an action into a habit, according to the University College London[1] *(Side note: Now you know why The Cheer Diet was specifically chosen as a 60 day plan versus some other random number).*

Before I show you how to overcome the two hurdles that allow us to form new habits, it's important to understand how and why humans form them in the first place.

The simplest answer is this: to prevent our brains from going into a state of overwhelm. You see, life can get pretty complicated and so we need quick, reliable ways to turn such complexities into something manageable.

For example, can you imagine if every few seconds you had to consciously think about controlling your breathing? Try it: Take a deep breath in through your nose, then out through your mouth. Now actively concentrate on this rhythm for the rest of your life.

Or how about blinking? In fact, give it a shot – try and take control over this bodily function: close and open your eye lids every few seconds for the next minute. I think you'll agree, consciously doing all this for the rest of your life sounds about as appealing as getting a wedgie in the middle of a full-out practice.

To be honest, just thinking about having to think about constantly breathing and blinking is making me nauseous. So the point is, if our body didn't automate most of the processes we need on a daily basis, our brains would literally get overloaded and fry. And the reason for this, is that it doesn't have that much conscious capacity – or in other words, **willpower**.

In fact, a very interesting research experiment showed that willpower is a finite resource[2,4] - you only get so much of it every day, and once it's gone, there's a very strong chance that your body will go into auto-pilot.

Listed below is a recap of the experiment, along with the results that were found according to the American Psychological Association:

"A scientist named Roy Baumeister brought subjects into a room, where the table before them held a plate of fresh-baked cookies and a bowl of radishes. Some subjects were asked to sample the cookies, while others were asked to eat the radishes. Afterward, they were given 30 minutes to complete a difficult geometric puzzle. Baumeister and his colleagues found that people who ate radishes (and resisted the enticing cookies) gave up on the puzzle after about 8 minutes, while the lucky cookie-eaters persevered on for nearly 19 minutes, on average. Drawing on willpower to resist the cookies, it seemed, drained the subjects' self-control for subsequent situations."

This explains why your body builds habits to try and automate everything – it wants to save willpower for times where you really need it (such as remembering the counts to your routine!)

It's also the reason why you automatically end up reaching for something to eat when your stomach starts growling, or worse, for sugar and caffeine when you start to feel tired. These actions aren't something you take consciously; they're habitual patterns which you've unknowingly trained yourself with.

So How Do We Break The Bad Habits?

Well *technically* speaking, we can't.

Once habits are in place, they become strong neurological connections in your brain, and unless there's some laser-precise brain surgery involved, those connections are here to stay.

However, what you *can* do is replace your old bad habits with even stronger new habits that provide the following two benefits:

1) Give you the reward you originally got from your old habit
2) Lead you into getting the results you want

It's like fighting a sumo wrestler with an even bigger sumo wrestler. So the obvious question is: what is it going to take to form newer, stronger habits?

The first thing you need to understand, is how habits actually form. Once you know their basic structure, and have the willpower needed, you can build as many new habits as you want.

Here's what happens: first there's a cue (or a trigger) which acts as the spark which sets everything off. When this cue or trigger is fired, you perform the action (or sequence of actions). Once this sequence is complete, you obtain some type of reward[5]. The reward is actually the whole reason behind why habits form in the first place. Think about it:

Nail biters get pleasure and satisfaction from the nibbling.

Smokers get an energized buzz (or high) from the nicotine.

Those who are addicted to working out get a rush of endorphins, which makes them feel good.

A dog does tricks because it knows you'll either give it some type of treat or affection ("good boy!").

As you can see, without a reward the habit would never form; it would just be a one-time action, never to be repeated again. But if you really want to make a lasting change, you need to understand all three phases of a habit and *when* to manipulate them. Let's take a look at an example of a young cheerleader called Mary.

The first thing Mary does upon waking up is have a glass of milk with a plate full of cookies. She's been doing this for the past five years. Can you spot the cue, the action and the reward in her habit? Think about it for a minute, then write down your answers below:

Cue:

Action:

Reward:

Hopefully, your answers are similar to mine: the cue was waking up, the action was eating simple carbohydrates, and the reward was that it kills the feeling of hunger while providing a sugar rush that makes her feel awake.

If Mary wanted to curb this habit, what could she do? We know that she can't just get rid of it – the connections in her brain have been made. But what if she were to modify it? Her cue of waking up is not going anywhere, this is obvious since everyone needs to sleep and thus, everyone will wake up. So the cue stays the same.

Now let's take a look at the reward, because once we understand this, we can put a sequence of actions in place that Mary can use.

She needs something that will kill the feeling of hunger after a long night of sleeping, so how about a vegetable omelette, an apple, and half a cup of coffee?

The protein from the eggs will keep her feeling fuller for longer while the apple and the cup of coffee can provide her with a quick burst of energy that she needs to function in the morning. While eating this way for the first week may be slightly challenging for Mary, it'll be heckuva lot more manageable then ditching breakfast completely.

Making subtle changes like the ones listed above involves minimal willpower, but can give you maximum results (addressing the second hurdle I was talking about when you want to change habits). Does all of this make sense? I hope so, because the problem with most diets and nutrition plans is that they take your current habits and try to completely replace all of them at once.

As you can probably imagine, this doesn't last and leads people to "yo-yo" or "rebound" on their diet plan; leaving them fatter, more miserable versions of themselves. We humans just don't have the willpower capacity to handle such massive and multiple changes all at once.

Fortunately, in *The Cheer Diet*, you'll be taking habits you already have (such as eating before practice, or eating after practice etc.) and modifying them ever-so-gently that it seems natural. Once these "gentle habits" have been worked on, only then will we completely replace them with ones which are more efficient.

"Hold on a second coach, I understand that it takes some willpower to change habits, but if it's is a limited resource, does that mean I'm screwed once I run out of it? Isn't there a way to increase it?"

Well actually, yes there is! In fact, there are two known ways to increase your willpower, and by design, each of them are built right into *The Cheer Diet*. Let's take a look at them, shall we?

First Way: Make It Grow

While your willpower is indeed limited, haven't you ever wondered why certain individuals seem to have more of it than others? Well that's because willpower is also like a muscle - it gets fatigued when you work it really hard, but it also becomes stronger once it has recovered.

The more you consciously stress your willpower, the stronger it gets, until the action you're expending energy on becomes (you guessed it) – *a habit!*

There will be times where you will really need to test your ability to resist temptations in the next 60 days. I hope you're ready, because the results are worth it, and you'll only come out stronger.

Actually, in a very odd way, the more good habits you can put in place, the easier it becomes to add *even more* good habits down the road because your willpower is constantly being challenged, and thus, constantly increasing. Win-Win!

Finally, there is one other (much faster) way to replenish your willpower...

Second Way: Your Diet

Research has shown that the brains in humans and animals (such as dogs) consume more energy (glucose) when they're active (consciously using up willpower) than when they're at rest (not doing much thinking.)[3]

In fact, as an organ, your brain is very energy-hungry. So it's no surprise that replenishing any lost glucose which your brain uses up will give you a quick mental boost[3].

But as we know with any sugar high, there is always a crash, and the benefits are short-lived. This is why in *The Cheer Diet*, you'll be eating foods that keep your blood sugar levels stable, so you can avoid major crashes and give your willpower a quick recharge on days your mental "gas tank" is running low.

Let's take a moment to do a quick recap everything you've just learnt:

- Our brains form habits to automate repetitive tasks and conserve willpower
- You cannot break old habits, only replace them with new ones
- It takes an average of 66 days to produce a new habit
- Every habit contains 3 main elements: the cue, the sequence of actions, and the reward
- The biggest hurdle you'll face when it comes to changing habits, is a lack of willpower
- Willpower is like a muscle – it gets fatigued, but can also be trained to become stronger over time
- To change a habit, understand the cue (what sets it off), then understand the reward (why you're doing it) then pick a sequence of actions that require the least amount of willpower to pull off.
- Trying to change every aspect of a habit is a recipe for disaster
- Willpower can be partially replenished through a good diet

The Habit Building Guide

To make sure that you have a high success rate while following *The Cheer Diet*, the first phase of the plan will revolve around your current eating cues. So for example, if you constantly find yourself in the middle of a drive-through window after practice, we won't change the fact that you like to eat after practice, only *what* you should be eating (basically, we just want to change your sequence of actions).

So the first thing we need to do, is to find your cues. For the next 7 days, use the Habit Cue Log I've provided in the next few pages to write down when and what you eat on a daily basis. (If you don't want to use the pages in this book, the log can also be downloaded and printed off from *The Cheer Diet* resource page here: http://bit.ly/cheerfiles - the password is **tcd2015**)

If you do this right, you will most likely see a pattern emerge. Once we have a pattern, we can work with it instead of *against it*.

How it works: Each table is to be used for a particular day of the week, and all you have to do is be aware of when you *feel* the need to eat. Then before actually eating, write down the time and try and pin point your actual cue. Be sure to log this using a **pencil** – you'll soon see why.

Finding the real cue can be tricky as there can be a whole bunch of factors that fire off your hunger signals such as: time of day, aromas, peer pressure, curiosity etc., but try your best. You don't have to over-think this.

Below is an example log for what a couple of days would look like. Just remember, while this is an example, it's not the definition of a **good** example because the foods being eaten aren't close to ideal. We'll get to what foods you *should* be eating soon.

Habit Cue Log [Example]

Day: Monday

Time	Cue	Meal
8am	Empty stomach/growling	Bowl of cereal
12pm	Lunch period bell rings	Chicken fingers and fries with bottle of gatorade
4pm	Turn on tv to watch my favourite show – need munchies	Microwaveable popcorn
5:30pm	Mom calls for dinner before cheer practice	Chicken pasta with garlic bread

Day: Tuesday

Time	Cue	Meal
8:20 am	Feeling of hunger	Leftover pizza and coffee
12pm	Lunch period bell rings	Burger with fries and a diet coke
3pm	Walking into Starbucks after school – the smell of coffee	A brownie and Grande Caramel Macchiato
6pm	Mom calls for dinner	Meat loaf and apple pie
10pm	Dorito TV Commercial	Half a bag of all dressed chips

Habit Cue Log

Day:

Time	Cue	Meal

Day:

Time	Cue	Meal

Day:

Time	Cue	Meal

Day:

Time	Cue	Meal

Day:

Time	Cue	Meal

Day:

Time	Cue	Meal

Day:

Time	Cue	Meal

Day:

Time	Cue	Meal

Optimizing Your Cues

Once you've filled out the Habit Cue Log, you should have an idea of when and why you eat at the certain times that you do. Hopefully, by putting some thought into your logs, you may have realized that your cues aren't always what you thought they were.

As an example, back when I was in school I always thought I ate lunch because that's just what everyone did at 12pm. Turns out my "cue" was meeting up at my friend's locker where we would inevitably talk about what we felt like eating that day, and end up in the cafeteria line-up. But if I ever skipped this cue and say, went to the library to sign out a new book, I never really felt hungry or compelled to eat... even if I met up with my friends later at a table where they were eating.

My cue was more social than anything else. On the other hand, I always thought that bed time was a cue. So whenever I felt like it was time to get some shut-eye, I would eat beforehand. Turns out that wasn't true at all. You see, I used to go to the gym every day, and I'm someone that doesn't like working out when it's crowded so I used to go late. It was the workout that had me wanting food – it just happened to be close to my bed time. On days where I couldn't manage to go to the gym and get my workout in for whatever reason, I wouldn't feel like eating before sleeping.

As you can see, it's easy to get confused as to what the real cue was. Because of this, I'd like you to take 10 minutes to go over your log and to make sure your cues are accurate. Do you eat lunch at 12pm because of the time itself, or because of some other factor? If the time is the factor than it shouldn't matter where you are – at school, at home, or at a job, because when 12pm hits, you should feel like eating. If you don't, your cue is probably not time based.

I cannot stress enough how important it is to spend some time on your cues, and making sure they're as accurate as can be. Your success depends on it.

Chapter 3: The Fundamentals Of Nutrition

A Food Pyramid That Actually Makes Sense

If you're a South Park fan, you may remember a parody they did about the American food pyramid a while back. For those that never watched it, here's how it all went:

The scene begins inside the USDA headquarters, where everyone is freaking out about dinner time that's fast approaching. It seems they're under a lot of pressure to deliver a magical solution that families can use to make healthier choices... or else they will die, apparently.

Nothing's seems to be working. Then, Cartman calls in and says how the answer is *"in the food pyramid"*

The head scientist is quick to confirm, *"The pyramid doesn't work! We've already tried it."* (which, humorously enough, is absolutely true - the traditional pyramid sucks)

Then Cartman lays the bombshell, *"...it's upside down!"*

The head scientist, desperate for a quick solution, orders his team to flip the pyramid. One of his colleagues seems absolutely shocked by this and says, *"You can't be serious! That would put butter and fat at the top..."*

"JUST FLIP THE DAMN PYRAMID!" the head scientist yells. And so they do, placing fats & oils as the top priority, followed by meat & dairy, fruits & vegetables, and lastly, grains. Magically, the computer simulations confirm the action, and past problems are suddenly solved. One scientist yells out, *"Sir, we've got a match!"*, while another says *"the nutrition is stabilizing!"* (not sure what that means but I laughed)

The scene cuts to everyone cheering, as dinner time in America has been saved.

Amidst the celebrations, the head scientist goes to one of his colleagues and says, *"Get the president on the phone... tell him to have some steak, with his butter."*

The end. (you can watch the video by going to TCD resource page: http://bit.ly/cheerfiles - password is **tcd2015**)

While South Park is obviously a cartoon that is fictional, in this instance what makes this skit absolutely hilarious (at least to those in the nutrition field) is that if they did flip the food pyramid like this, people would definitely be better off. John Vorhaus, author of *The Comic Toolbox* once said that *"Comedy is truth and pain."*

That statement has never been truer. But while the South Park food pyramid is a step in the right direction, I'm going to present a food pyramid that is backed a mountain of scientific evidence. What makes my pyramid so awesome?

Well instead of telling you which specific foods to eat and prioritize, it showcases all of the major components of nutrition, and stacks them in order or importance. This will allow you to easily create any meal plan your heart desires.

On the next page, you'll see what this pyramid looks like, and each layer will be explained in detail. Let's start with the base of the pyramid which contains the most important component: calories!

Calories

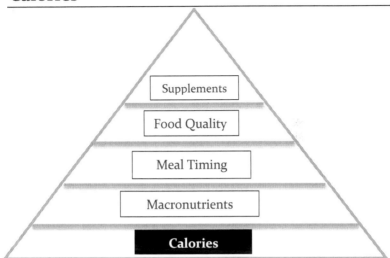

Ah, calories. They're quite possibly the most misunderstood form of measurement, yet at the same time, they've become the most popular noun that the mainstream media uses to discuss anything related to nutrition.

Here's what I find fascinating: everyone knows that a food item which contains hundreds and hundreds of calories is bad for you. You'll hear the major news channels scream at the top of their lungs about how a Frappuccino containing 400 calories is absolutely absurd, especially when you drink it alongside an actual meal.

It seems everywhere you look, low calorie options are the perfect way for people to justify their crappy eating habits (Diet coke and a side order of nachos layered with trans-fats, anyone?)

On the other hand, whenever I'm trying to give nutrition advice, the one thing no one ever wants to do, is keep track of their caloric intake.

In fact, it seems that counting calories is considered an act of social suicide. Yet, the millions of people who are on Weight Watchers™ will happily tally up their "points" so they can lose weight. That's like saying, *"Instead of counting dollars, I'm going to keep track of my pennies."*

Wow, what a brilliant idea! *cough*

It doesn't matter how you spin it, market it, slice it or twist it, the amount of calories that you consume will be one of the biggest factors that contribute to your diet's success – regardless if that diet is designed to help you lose weight, gain weight, stay the same or improve performance. The secret, of course, is in knowing exactly how much.

This is not just a statement, or something I'm taking an educated guess on, **this is law** (specifically, the 1st law of thermodynamics).

Not All Calories Are Created Equal

When I inform my clients about this fact, their initial reaction is always followed by some type of smart ass comment such as, *"So you're saying I can eat only Oreos, but as long as I watch how many calories I'm taking in, I can get the results I want?"*

Obviously not – a calorie from a cookie isn't worth nearly as much to us athletes as a calorie from, say, brown rice or chicken[1].

If you'll recall from chapter 1, a calorie is basically a unit of energy, and it can be used by your body to perform a whole list of functions.

Obviously, the primary function that we're concerned with is fuel for your muscles to increase performance and speed up recovery. Any excess calories which are circulating in your system, are stored for later use in the form of fat. There is no exception to this rule.

The 3 Sates Of The Human Body

Depending on how many calories you consume, your body will respond by being in one of the following three states listed below. Remember, it is physiologically *impossible* for your body to be in more than one of these states at a time – anyone who tries to convince you otherwise is either trying to sell you lies, or is just plain misinformed.

State 1: Negative Calorie Balance

Simply put, this is when you're burning off more calories than you're taking in. Regardless of the quality of the food, if more is being burnt off than taken in, weight loss will eventually occur. Let's go back to the cheeky Oreo comment for a second. You might be wondering if it's possible to be in a negative calorie balance by eating junk.

The answer, as we saw in chapter one, is a obviously "yes". But the problem is that junk food is generally high in sodium and low in protein, so the water retention and/or bloating will usually cover up the loss of something you don't want: muscle tissue.

Remember, being in a negative calorie balance doesn't necessarily mean that your body will only target fat cells to burn energy from – it can also take the energy it needs by sacrificing muscle tissue (something we *really* don't want).

State 2: Neutral Calorie Balance (BMR)

A neutral balance is achieved when you're burning off everything you're taking in. The amount of calories you take in during a neutral balance is known as your BMR (Basal Metabolic Rate). This means you're not gaining weight, nor losing it. After my personal clients go through a successful dieting phase, and are happy with their results, helping them hit their BMR is usually the next step in the process. This allows them to keep what they've achieved, and not "yo-yo."

State 3: Positive Calorie Balance

Here it is - the primary reason the entire world is getting fat. You can't blame sugar, or alcohol, or wheat, or dairy, or any other type of food or substance. The simple fact of the matter is, when more calories are taken in than burnt off, bodyweight goes up. This is also known as a hypercaloric diet. From experience, 99% of women want to avoid being in this state, while most guys I know will want to do nothing *but* stay in it.

The reason? A hypercaloric diet is the only reliable way to build muscle and get bigger. Even for guys that are supposedly "juicing", being in a positive calorie balance is required – because if they weren't, all the juice in the world wouldn't help them get jacked up. I say this to illustrate how important these 3 phases are, not to condone any steroid or substance use.

Finally, before I wrap up this section, I want you to accept one very important fact of life: **you can never improve what you don't measure.**

It doesn't matter what you're keeping track of – your calories, your weight, your waist to hip ratio, the number of stars on your Starbucks card or even the amount of AirMiles™ you've accumulated, you will always be dealing with some type of number which will either be **increasing, decreasing or staying the same**.

The trick is to find the right type of number to measure, make the process dead simple to accomplish, and then use the data to help improve your life and/or get you closer to your goals.

This is why you don't have to count calories on *The Cheer Diet*. Not because it isn't important, but because I'll be giving you a more important number to keep track of while the expertly crafted recipes and habit loops we create will always keep your caloric intake on track (more on that later). Now let's move on to the 2nd most important component: Macronutrients.

Macronutrients – What are they?

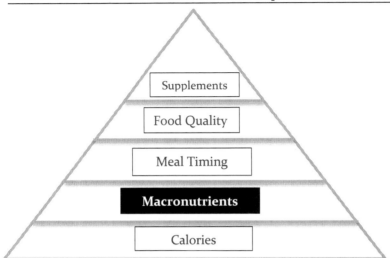

The standard definition states that *"macronutrients are nutrients that are needed by the body in large quantities"*. Some people tend to get confused when the word "macro" and "large quantities" are used in the same sentence, but what they are confusing it with is **micro**nutrients - which are needed by your body in small amounts.

So remember, macro = more, micro = less.

So what exactly are these nutrients that we need to consume in large quantities? Luckily, there are only three: Protein, Carbohydrates (Carbs) & Fats. We'll dive into each one so you can understand why they're needed by your body. Let's begin with the most important one for athletes.

Protein

Also known as polypeptides; they are found in the cells of all living things and are essential to health.

Most of the protein that is in our bodies is made up of about 20 different amino acids. This list of 20 is divided into two groups: **Essential Amino Acids** and **Nonessential Amino Acids.**

Essential amino acids must be taken in through diet because the body cannot synthesize them on its own. This is one of the major reasons I don't recommend going vegan; plants based foods are lacking essential amino acids while meat is a *complete* source of protein.

So shouldn't it make sense that we should eat both plants and animals? I think so. In fact, "vegan" was the term our ancient ancestors used to describe the village idiot who couldn't hunt or fish. True story. Probably.

While on one hand we have Essential amino acids, on the other we have Nonessential amino acids.

I personally hate these two terms because it makes it seem that one group is more important than the other, which is definitely not the case. The only reason the second group is called "non-essential" is because the body can synthesize these amino acids on its own. All 20 amino acids are important for optimal health, just remember that.

Carbohydrates (Carbs)

Oh boy, where do I even begin with carbs? It happens to be one of the most feared macronutrients, to the point where it seems like some people have a phobia of it (Carbophobia?)

Well I'm here to say that you don't need to fear carbs like most people do. What you really need do need to do, is figure out which types of carbs to eat, when to eat them, and in what quantities. Carbohydrates are the body's primary source of fuel - point blank period.

Let me go on a tangent for a second and take this fuel analogy a bit further - assume you have a car with a tank that can hold 50 liters of fuel. What happens when you try and pour in more than 50 liters? Well, either the gas pump will start to "click" or you'll experience the benefits of gasoline being sprayed all over your clothes.

Unfortunately (or fortunately) our bodies handle over-fueling a bit differently. As you know by now, it just stores the extra fuel for later use (in the form of fat). Looking at the general population, if the human stomach acted more like a solid gas tank, and its primary reaction was to make someone throw up every time they tried to over-fuel themselves, we wouldn't have an obesity problem.

This book would instead be called *The Confidence Diet: How to figure out your daily food requirements so you don't randomly throw up during competition.*

Alright enough talking about bodily fluids, let's get back on point. Here are the four types of carbohydrates which we need to be concerned with: Low Glycemic/High Glycemic and New Age/Old Age.

Low Glycemic/High Glycemic Carbohydrates

The Glycemic index, or GI, ranks carbohydrates according to their effect on our blood glucose levels. Foods that are low glycemic (such as oatmeal, brown rice, whole wheat etc.) cause low fluctuations in our blood glucose and insulin while foods that are high glycemic (sugar, fructose, white rice etc.) obviously do the opposite. It's those insulin levels that we as athletes will be focusing on.

New Age/Old Age Carbs

New age carbs refers to foods that we have been consuming for the past few thousand years such as rice, wheat, grains etc. Old age carbs are foods that our species have been consuming since we were cavemen... you know, a time where our language consisted of 15 random noises.

It was also a time when a man showed his affection for a woman by taking down a buffalo with a long pointy tree branch. But now, instead of taking down buffalos, apparently it's all about sliding into someone's DM. We sure have come a long way.

Fats

This is another macronutrient that is feared, and gets a bad reputation in my opinion. So what exactly is fat? Is it the bumpy cellulite you see on the overweight woman at the beach who can't pick her correct bikini size? Is it the white stuff surrounding your cut of Tbone steak? Or is it the liquid you use to cook your food with? The answer is obviously, "all of the above."

The actual scientific term for fat is **lipids,** as it's insoluble in water. Think of lips, then think of lids. Lipids, easy. There are 3 types of lipids that you need to know about for the first 10 seconds... after which you'll only need to know about one since it's the most important.

The 3 Types Of Lipids:

- **Triglycerides**
- **Phospholipids**
- **Sterols**

The one were concerned with are the triglycerides because they represent 95% of the fat we consume. Your body happens to store fat in the form of triglycerides as well. The saying "you are what you eat," definitely applies here. First, let's break down that long name as this will help you remember it better. Scientific names are usually logical so once you understand the logic, it will forever click in your brain (unless you hate science, which is seriously uncool).

The word begins with the letters "tri" meaning 3 (duh). This number represents the number of fatty acids, while the term "glyceride" refers to the 3 carbon atom backbone to which the fatty acids are attached to.

Below is a little illustration that will help you visualize it.

```
|G|====[Fatty Acid 1]==============
|L|
|Y|
|C|====[Fatty Acid 2]====
|E|
|R|
|O|
|L|====[Fatty Acid 3]=========
```

With me so far? Cool. Next thing you need to know is that the length of the fatty acid molecule isn't always the same. This is being accurately represented by the illustration above; fatty acid 1 is definitely the more dominant player out of the three.

Now, the chain length of the triglycerides are divided into three varieties. We have Short-Chain Fatty Acids, Medium-Chain Fatty Acids and Long-Chain Fatty Acids.

- **Short Chain** represents a fatty acid length of 6 carbon atoms or less
- **Medium Chain** represents a fatty acid length of 6-12 carbon atoms
- **Long Chain** represents a fatty acid length of 14 or more carbon atoms

Why are chain lengths important? Because it will determine the speed and method of digestion as well as the function of the fat you eat. More on which fats to eat will be discussed later.

Levels Of Saturation

Ok so we know that a triglyceride is a type of lipid and comes in three varieties: short chain, medium chain and long chain. But annoyingly, triglycerides can also be categorized by the type of carbon atom bonds found inside the fatty acid.

If the carbon atoms in a fatty acid is bonded together by single bonds only, we call that **saturated fat**. "What exactly is it saturated by", you ask?

Hydrogen!

Every carbon atom in that chain has 2 hydrogen atoms attached to it, for company. Some would say cheerleaders are usually saturated with glitter. As you can see in the diagram below, saturated fat forms a very neat and clean looking molecule... this means that a bunch of them could be packed tightly together resulting in solids at room temperature. Think butter and lard. But it's not always a solid, there are a few exceptions such as coconut oil and palm kernel oil.

```
     H HHH
     | | | |
H-O-C-C-C-C-H
     | | | |
     H HHH
```

However, if the fatty acid chain has two carbon atoms that are attached together by a double bond, it's called **mono-unsaturated fat**. Mono refers to the number of double bonds in the entire chain (one) and it's unsaturated because at the carbon double bond location, it's not hosting as many hydrogen atoms as saturated fat.

```
     H H    H
     | |    |
... -C-C= C-C- ...
     |    | |
     H    H H
```

Still with me? Good.

The diagram above represents the double-bond section of this particular fatty acid molecule. The shape of a monounsaturated molecule isn't as neat as saturated fat.

If you were playing Tetris, this molecule would be like the annoying "Z" block that's a pain in the behind to slot away neatly. And as such, at room temperature, it's found in the form of liquids (olive oil, canola oil etc.)

And finally we have a third type of triglyceride called **poly-unsaturated fat**. "Poly" because it's got more than one double bond, and "unsaturated" because just like monounsaturated fat, it can't host too many hydrogen atoms at its double bond locations (See diagram below). Again, just like with monounsaturated fat this molecule has a messy shape, and therefore comes in the form of liquids. Alpha Linoleic acid is one example, while other oils include cottonseed, corn and safflower.

```
    HH    H
    | |   |
... -C-C=C-C-C=C ...
    |   | | | |
    H   HHH H
```

Piecing The Fat Puzzle Together

The final thing you need to know is that foods rarely contain *one* type of triglyceride. They all contain a mix of everything you've read above. For example, butter is 65% saturated fat, 31% monounsaturated fat and 4% polyunsaturated fat. But because the majority of its construction at a molecular level is saturated, it stays solid at room temperature - and even more so when you put it in the fridge, at which point it won't spread nicely on your toast. Don't holes in your toast totally piss you off? Yeah, me too.

On the flipside we have olive oil which contains 14% saturated fat, 74% monounsaturated fat and 10% polyunsaturated fat which is why it's a liquid. Also, for future reference I'll be using acronyms when talking about the different type of triglycerides to make things easier. They are listed below - get to know them as well as your cheer routine.

SFA = Saturated Fatty Acid
MUFA = Monounsaturated Fatty Acid
PUFA = (...take a wild guess; consider it a pop quiz)

So why did I bother with such an exhaustive overview on fat? Because the biggest fear most people have is that if you *eat* fat, you'll *get* fat, but you now know from chapter 1 that this is definitely not true.

What you need to be concerned with is the types of dietary fats you consume, and that's about it. There are good fats and bad fats. Good fats such as Omega-3/6/9 fatty acids, polyunsaturated and monounsaturated fats are more beneficial than saturated and trans fats. Having said that, don't think that I'm telling you to completely cut out saturated fats because in moderation it has a specific job to do. Trans fatty acids from natural animal meat is not something you need to fear. It's the hydrogenated garbage in things such as potato chips you need to avoid.

Also, good sources of natural saturated fat such as butter, is actually good for you. Butter tastes awesome, why would you completely avoid it? Now here's a little trick, look into consuming fats that are known as medium-chain-triglycerides (MCT's). The beauty of MCT's is that in about a few hours after ingestion, they are readily available to the tissues in your body (such as muscles) as fuel. Also, from what I've experienced and read, they are hardly ever *stored* as fat in your body!

MCT's also spare protein, which means when you are cutting down on carbs, your body won't be eyeing your muscles as a fuel source. This is very crucial to our goals because remember - we want to lose fat, have more energy while minimizing muscle loss. Google MCT oils if you want to try some or just use coconut oil.

Meal Timing

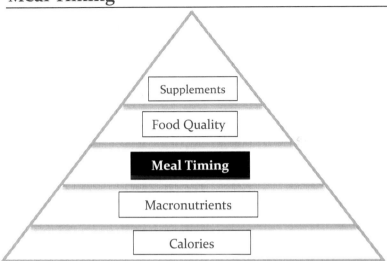

As you can clearly see based on my pyramid, timing your food intake isn't as high a priority as some make it out to be. In fact there are many health "gurus" and nutrition "experts" that say that if you eat carbs during the evening or god forbid, before bed time, you'll wake up looking like Honey Booboo. Too bad they don't have any evidence to back this claim.

This whole *"don't eat carbs at night"* has become repeated so often that it has now achieved myth status - one I was planning on debunking in the first chapter. But since meal timing is part of the pyramid, I had to save it for this section.

So how did this recommendation gain popularity in the first place? And is there any logic behind it?

Well, yes. It was thought that when you're awake and doing stuff (like training, walking around the mall etc.) that your metabolism is running in a faster gear, thus you'll be burning more calories than when you're asleep and completely immobile.

Sounds reasonable enough, doesn't it? In fact, there was a study[2] which looked at 12 individuals and their metabolic activity during sleep, and it did find this to be true. Here's a quote: *"Energy expenditure decreased during the **first half** of the night, reached a nadir (a 35% decrease)"*

A 35% decrease is definitely substantial, and enough to scare people into starving themselves before bed time. But the key here is that the drop was noticed only in first half of the night. What about the other half? Well let's dig further:

*"...On the other hand, carbohydrate oxidation showed **no remarkable changes** from the onset of sleep but began to increase before awakening."*

Isn't that interesting? Not only did the ability to burn carbs at night **not** show much change, it actually *increased* during morning time. Finally, the researchers also found that as the subjects hit a deeper level of sleep (called RMR, or rapid eye movement), their metabolism shot right back up again. This rise and fall meant the body's average metabolic rate over the course of the night *hardly* changed.

Now remember, that data is just for the average person. Allstar cheerleaders aren't average, they're serious performance athletes – and things look even brighter for such a group of individuals! There was one study[3] which I found even more interesting because they found out the following: *"To conclude, prolonged exercise repeated for 4 days was associated with **increases** in SHR (sleeping heart rate) and SMR (sleeping metabolic rate) during the night following each day of exercise concomitantly with an enhanced lipid (fat) oxidation."*

What does this mean? Well unless you are very obese, or someone that doesn't move very much, not only does your metabolism **not** slow down during sleep, it actually *increases* so you can burn more fat! So instead of avoiding food at night, maybe what we all should be doing after a hard practice, is eating *more* of it.

As you can probably tell, that's not just a random guess I pulled out of thin air. It seems science has, once again, proven that turning conventional wisdom on its head is a very good idea. Here's what I mean:

There was a study[4] done in 1997 which took 10 women, divided them into two groups (AM group and a PM group) and fed them two meals per day; breakfast and lunch. For 6 weeks straight, the AM group ate about 70% of their daily calories during breakfast while the PM group obviously took in their 70% during the evening.

After the 6 weeks were up, they swapped the groups so now the AM group became the PM group, and the PM group became the AM group. They then implemented the whole morning/evening protocol for another 6 weeks.

At the end of this 15 week study (3 weeks were used as a stabilization period), the results were rather interesting: On average, the AM group lost more weight than the PM group, however the PM group lost more *fat mass* than the AM group. Basically, those that ate a heavy breakfast and a light dinner ended up losing fat as well as muscle mass (not good), but those that ate light in the mornings but heavy in the evenings lost mainly fat (this is what we want).

The take home point is that if you have control over when you eat your meals, you are better off stuffing your face at night, since our goal is to maximize muscle to keep you strong, while getting rid of any excess baggage that you don't need to carry around.

But on the other hand, if you can't eat heavier meals at night for whatever reason, don't sweat your cheerbow over it because as long as the first two bases of your pyramid are covered, you'll still see fantastic results.

That's enough talk about sleep, what about eating before and after practice? Does this matter?

Absolutely. Knowing how to fuel yourself around your training schedule is the *only* time you should be worried about the timing of your food, because it actually has a direct impact on your performance. The reason I spent the previous 3 pages on night time eating, is to show you how negligible it really is.

Pre & Post Training Nutrition

To understand which foods you should eat around training time, you need to have a basic understanding of digestion. The reason? It's not just about the foods you eat that matters, it's about what your body *absorbs*.

Here's how it works: When you eat, the food sits in your stomach where the acids break it down into something your body can actually use. It then travels into your intestines (first small, then large). Now, your intestines are where all the magic happens, as that's where most of your absorption takes place. Humans are actually very efficient and usually absorb upwards of 90% of the foods we eat. After the intestines, whatever is left unabsorbed gets eliminated as waste. Also note that women, on average, take longer to digest foods than men do[5].

So before you start training, what we want to consume are foods that meet the following criteria:

1. Leave the stomach quickly
2. Absorbed in the intestines where it can enter your bloodstream as useable fuel as quickly as possible.

And generally speaking, there are only 2 types of foods that meet our criteria: simple carbohydrates (HG) and whey protein.

As you'll remember from the macronutrient section, there are two types of carbohydrates that you need to concern yourself with as an athlete: Low glycemic (LG) and high glycemic (HG).

The secret lies in knowing which type of carbohydrate to eat and at what times in order to maximize performance. For example, eat HG carbs at the wrong time, and you'll crash by the time practice even begins. Eat LG carbs at the wrong time, and they simply won't be absorbed quickly enough, and will just sit in your intestines making you feel bloated and slow.

To prevent such things from happening, take a look at the graph below:

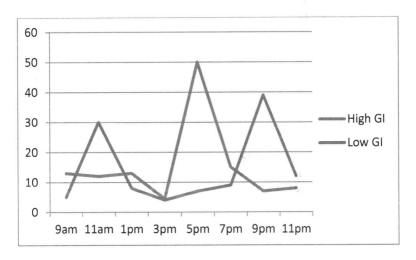

This graph showcases the carb intake of a cheerleader who has practice coming up at 6pm (she also read *The Cheer Diet* because she's a smart cookie). The left axis represents the amount of carbs eaten (in grams), while the bottom axis represents the time of day.

First, let's take a look at the blue line (if you're reading a printed version of this book, that's the High GI line, which has the biggest mountain). The type of HG carb she consumed doesn't matter, but for the sake of entertainment, let's assume it was a Boston Cream donut. Yum.While a majority of the population would look down on a serious athlete choosing a donut over something like white rice, you have to realize that at the end of the day, your body doesn't care where the glucose molecule came from – it'll absorb it just the same.

You'll notice that throughout the day, the amount of HG carbs were low; the minor amounts you see on the graph could be sources such as sugar in the morning coffee, condiments on her scrambled eggs etc. But an hour before practice, at 5pm, she had a huge 50 gram surge of HG carbs.

The reason is simple - it almost guarantees that the sugar in the donut (combined with adequate water intake) will be available as useable fuel to power through the jumps, tumbling and stunting sections of her routine. And let's be real, carbs from a donut are a lot more delicious than carbs from rice.

However, if this cheerleader had practice at 9pm, can you see why she would crash? Simple sugars can be absorbed and enter your bloodstream within the hour, and if you don't do something to use it up, your body will have no choice but to store it as fat. (remember, 1st law of thermodynamics states that energy cannot be created nor destroyed, therefor it *must* go somewhere).

Now let's take a look at the Low GI line on the graph (the one with two peaks).

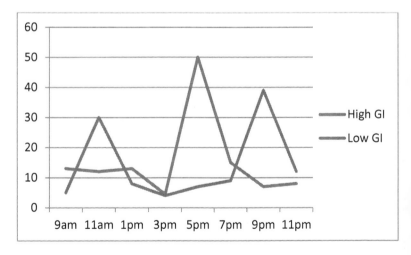

Let's assume her LG carb of choice were steel cut oats and brown rice. As you can see, she started off her day with the oatmeal – a solid choice as it takes a few hours to digest, is a decent source of fiber, and will provide her with a steady stream of energy to get her through her school day.

Then after practice, she likely had some grilled chicken with a bowl of brown rice. Why did she choose LG carbs instead of HG after her practice? Because she knows she won't be active anymore, and the last thing you want is for all those carbs to rush into your bloodstream while you're at home, hibernating on the couch to another episode of *The Walking Dead*.

Now I will say that if post practice you don't have access to quality LG carbs, then HG carbs can be an *ok* choice since your metabolic rate will still be in high gear (assuming you weren't lazy and busted your behind at practice).

The graph you saw showed just one example of how a cheerleader can time her food intake intelligently. If she wasn't able to eat an hour before practice, the smart thing to do would be to have her oatmeal or brown rice a few hours prior (around 3-4pm) so that by the time practice hits, there would be useable fuel in her bloodstream.

To make things easy, in the recipe section of the book you'll find smoothies and meals that have been specifically designed to help fuel you before practice.

Food Quality

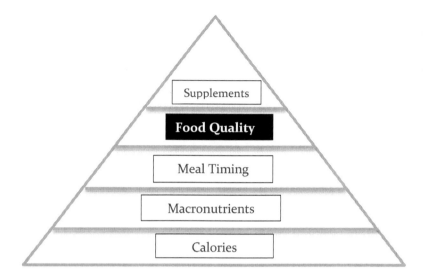

I'm not going to spend too much time on this section since I already made a case for organic food earlier, so I'm sure you have a general idea of what to expect. But beyond that, I should say that constantly eating "clean" as a way of life is a joke – and this statement is coming from someone who's gotten his clients down to single digit body fat levels, on multiple occasions, and never had to make them give up foods like ice cream, fast food or even beer. And no, their cholesterol and blood pressure levels weren't in any type of danger. In fact, they were all perfectly healthy.

So what exactly is *clean* eating?

Well, it definitely doesn't involve washing your food with Windex, I can tell you that. Usually, people who've joined this "clean eating" movement avoid any and all foods that come in boxes, from a fast food joints, or aren't in a form that nature intended. While there's nothing wrong with it, for me, it's a little too extremist in nature.

I'll use organic produce over any genetically modified counterpart to make my fruit smoothies all day, but that doesn't mean I don't enjoy Nutella or a bowl of Cinnamon Toast Crunch once in a while. In fact, if you follow the *The Cheer Diet* the way I've outlined it, you'll be getting your veggies, meats and other quality foods anyways, so going out of your way to eat "clean" is hardly necessary.

This might sound hypocritical, but it really isn't as long as the first two bases of the pyramid aren't violated. If you think about it, Cheerleading as a sport is a perfect example of blending multiple disciplines in one – you can't just be a tumbler, or just a jumper. You can definitely specialize, but you still have to practice all the elements in order to put out a routine that wins.

Similarly, there's no reason to belong to certain "nutritional camps" such as raw food, vegan, paleo, low carb, clean etc. Do you know who follows these micro-cults? Those that don't know any better; or those that like to inconvenience themselves for no apparent reason; or those that don't have any friends (oh snap!)

I'm joking, of course. Plenty of people get through life by eating clean 24/7, but I'm here to make sure what you eat increases performance, not inconveniences you. **Bottom Line?** Here's a chain of command to follow if you really care about quality: Go organic and use the recipes in this book whenever possible. If organic is too financially taxing, stick to whole foods (meats, eggs, veggies, fruits etc.) If that's not possible, try buying quality meals that have been freshly prepared by restaurants. Next up in line are your supplements such as protein shakes, meal replacement bars etc. Below that you have you fast food joints, which still offer halfway decent meals if you skip the fries and opt for a salad. Finally, in last place you have your KD and TV dinners. Yuck.

Trust me, spending any more time that this on food quality is a real waste of your life (and willpower). Instead, why not use it to become a better cheerleader? ☺

It's time to move on to the final piece of the puzzle: **supplements.**

Supplements

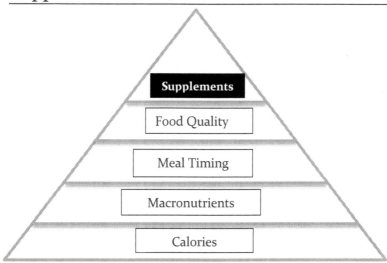

Ah, supplements. The multi-billion dollar industry that I've decided to slot away into a tiny corner at the top of my pyramid. Now you may be thinking, *"Coach, if supplements are so insignificant, why are they marketed so heavily?"*

Good question! It's because you cannot sell "eat less calories" as a pill. But as soon as you can, you can bet your tube of glitter that they'll try and market the heck out of it.

Now I'd like you to know something - while I'm not going to be talking about any scary, illegal or shady compounds, I will say that if you're under 18, anything but a daily multivitamin and some whey protein powder is all you should ever consider taking.

Everything else that I've listed here is for older female athletes that want an edge. If you're not sure that a supplement is right for you, check with your doctor and make sure your parents know.

Whey protein

You already know what protein is from the macronutrient section of the book, so I won't spend much time going over the basics. All you need to know about whey is that it's a liquid by-product of cheese production, and is the fastest absorbing out of all other protein sources available today.

Most of the quality whey you can buy is also 20-25% BCAA's (Branched Chain Amino Acids). Whey protein is the reason I think people who pay for pure BCAA's are complete dorks. There is no need! BCAA's are already in whey protein which happens to be reasonably priced, and if you buy the right formula and/or flavor, it can be a delicious treat to boot. Pure BCAA's on the other hand, usually aren't (with the exception of Xtend^{TM} which tastes decent). In my world, it's all about getting the biggest bang for your buck. Now you should know that there are a bunch of different types of whey proteins (Whey isolate, whey concentrate, whey hydrolysate etc.) and each have their pros and cons. Isolate yields the most amount of protein per scoop and is so pure, those that are lactose intolerant shouldn't have any problems taking it (I'd still double check with your doctor).

Concentrate is the cheapest of them all but can sometimes cause bloating if you buy the *really* cheap stuff. Also, lots of Chinese manufacturers have known to sell their concentrate formulas with cheap sugar fillers, so be careful. Then there's Hydrolsate which absorbs the quickest. Which one should you buy? Whichever floats your boat. I usually go for isolate but at times I also buy "blends" which contain all three. Check the label and make sure you're getting *at least* 23g of protein per 30g scoop – that's a solid range.

The brand I trust hands down is ON (Optimum Nutrition) – test after test, when stacked up against other products, independent labs have found them to be far superior. You cannot go wrong with that award-winning brand (P.S I'm *not* being paid to say that either). More info: http://thecheerdiet.com/links/protein/

Multivitamin

Cheap, effective and can take care of any holes in your diet plan. A multivitamin is the shotgun in your nutritional tool box. If you follow the nutritional guidelines and food list I've provided, then you probably won't need it. But it's better to be safe than sorry.

I don't care what you buy nor from who you buy. Indulge your inner child and buy the gummy multivitamins like I do at times. You can get your candy fix and daily micronutrients all in one go, so why wouldn't you?

Flintstones is another great option! However I will say that if you buy the really kiddy stuff, you should opt to double the dosage on training days. On every other day, follow the label guidelines.

One last tip: Liquid formulas are usually absorbed better and faster so if pills aren't your thing, then that's another great option for you.

Regardless of what delivery mechanism you choose, take it daily.

Vitamin D

Sunscreen, video games, smartphones and the rise of vampire culture are just a few of the reasons why the North American population is ridiculously deficient in Vitamin D. And this causes everyone to become miserable, fat and lethargic.

What's more, every part of your body needs Vitmain D for optimal functioning; without it, your metabolic rate will suffer, your energy levels will be low, insulin sensitivity will go out the window, you'll randomly feel hungry, and fat will infiltrate your muscles[5] like a group of NAVY Seals raiding a terrorist bunker.

Another problem seems to be that the general recommended daily dosage of Vitmain D is too low. So we have "experts" and "health organizations" which are telling people that they need X amount, when in reality they need about 5X or even 10X[6].

Having said all of that, know that taking Vitamin D doesn't affect fat loss directly - it's not a thermogenic compound like caffeine. If you take enough, what it will do is make sure that your body is functioning optimally so that you either return to your regular body fat levels, or have a much easier time losing fat when a proper plan is in place. It's like removing the monkey wrench stuck inside a giant malfunctioning machine, then greasing it – so it'll work as intended, but not much better.

Recommended Dosage: Depending on your activity levels, where you live (sunny or not so sunny) and how often you go outside, taking anywhere from 2000-4000 IU (international units) per day should be sufficient. You can even cycle it and take more on training days and less on rest days. Also, worrying about overdose is not an issue since like most people, you're probably deficient anyways, but try and stay under 5000-7000 IU per day.

More info: http://thecheerdiet.com/links/vitd

Fish oil

The list of benefits of fish oil are so vast, it comes across as the typical too-good-to-be-true scam. But luckily, it isn't. There's an absolute mountain of scientific data backing this supplement and it should be a staple for any athlete in my opinion – young or old, short or tall, new or experienced. If ever there was a substance that could do it all, I'd put my money on fish oils. However, on *The Cheer Diet*, here are some very specific reasons why we want to be taking fish oil:

1. It helps reduce muscle soreness[7]
2. Increases brain activity
3. Helps lower cortisol levels[9]
4. Improves joint function and mobility[8]

Recommended dose: If you're someone that is little (i.e short, light or generally a flyer) then 1 tbsp daily, for the rest of your life, is a good idea. If you're someone who's taller/larger/more muscular (such as a base and/or tumbler) then on rest days you should take 1 tbsp in the morning, and on training days you'll do the same but take another ½ tbsp with your post practice meal. If you're someone that regularly eats fish such as salmon, then ½ tbsp per day should be more than enough.

Try and take fish oil with food instead of by itself. Some might think that taking straight oil is weird, and it is if you buy cheap stuff. Personally, I recommend the brand called Ascenta, which sell lemon flavored fish oil that goes down with minimal fuss, especially when chased with some orange juice.

While gel capsules might sound easy and convenient, you'll need to take 5-7 of them just to equal 1 tbsp. Honestly, that's just a waste of time in my opinion. Holly has become a total champ at taking fish oils, and if she can manage it, trust me, so you can you ☺

More info: http://thecheerdiet.com/links/fishoil

Magnesium (Mg)

When you think of improving bone health, what is the one micronutrient that instantly comes to your mind?

Chances are, it's probably calcium. But calcium is just a small part of the equation. You see, it's actually **magnesium** that helps absorb the calcium and metabolize vitamin D, which is essential to the health of your bones and to prevent (or treat) osteoporosis.

In fact, magnesium is involved with around 300 different (and very vital) bodily functions such as: more restful sleep, helping the body burn fat, regulation of the nervous system and protein synthesis - which helps build muscle.

There are two standout studies which showcase the power of this forgotten micronutrient: In the first one[11], they compared three groups of people; group 1 did absolutely no training but received 10 mg of magnesium per kg of body weight, group 2 and 3 were active taekwondo practitioners but only group 2 got 10 mg per kg of bodyweight in magnesium. The results showed that group 2 had the highest natural testosterone production out of all three. In the other study[12], they took a group of 18-30 year olds and made them go through an intense leg strength training program. The only difference was that one group took 8 mg of magnesium per kilogram of body weight a day while the other group didn't. So what happened? Here's a quote:

"results indicated a significant increase for the M (mag) group compared to the C (control) group in absolute T, relative T adjusted for body weight (T/BWT), and relative T adjusted for lean body mass"

The "T" stands for testosterone and lean body mass, which means they likely put on muscle and burnt fat. Now as a young lady you may be thinking: *"Muscle mass? Strength training? Testosterone? I don't think I want to take magnesium... it'll turn me all manly!"*

But nothing could be further from the truth.

The testosterone increase is dependent on the natural processes and limits of *your* body – guys will obviously see a greater increase, but as a woman, your body does produce (and require) testosterone to function normally, just as men need a certain amount of estrogen.

The difference is, when you take magnesium and train hard, your natural levels of testosterone, which your body needs to function at its absolute peak, will be optimized. It certainly won't produce extra testosterone out of nowhere, so don't worry – your femininity is perfectly safe.

I think you get the picture by now – magnesium is not something you want to be deficient in, especially as an athlete. But unfortunately a deficiency in it is quite rampant.

Some experts say that up to 75% of Americans don't get enough[10] of this micronutrient, and the trend is similar for other Westernized countries as well.

I have to say that personally, the day I started supplementing with extra magnesium, I noticed a huge improvement in the quality of my sleep. Basically, I now sleep like a baby - as soon as my head hits the pillow, I'm out cold, and I love it.

Recommended dose: If you want to be ideal and base your dose on the studies, then aim to get around 4-5 mg per pound of bodyweight, per day. If you want to make things brain-dead easy, take an extra 400-500 mg of it on training days, since on rest days you'll get your magnesium from your multi and the foods you eat.

Truth be told, if you find that taking extra magnesium helps, then 500 mg a day on top of your multi should be just fine since the body can eliminate extra magnesium that is consumed. Magnesium overdose is rare but as I stated, it won't hurt to talk to your doctor.

More info: http://thecheerdiet.com/links/mag

Caffeine (From Coffee)

When I consult Powerlifters and MMA athletes on how to increase performance and improve their body composition, straight caffeine (in form of pills) is one of the most potent tools in the toolbox. However, as a young female cheerleader I cannot recommend you take synthesized (lab-created) caffeine. In fact, I'd say stay away from it for two reasons:

1. The diet itself along with the basic supplements I listed earlier should help your body be running in a peak state, so any extra energy from caffeine isn't necessary (you'll learn exactly how caffeine works in chapter 5).

2. If you do need a pick-me-up on a day you're feeling tired - the natural caffeine from coffee is vastly superior and safer for a young female adult. In fact, let's talk more about why coffee is awesome.

You see, there are two groups of people in this world; those that like coffee, and those that aren't people. Seriously, if water wasn't *absolutely* essential for my survival and wellbeing, coffee would top the list as my most consumed beverage. Yes, even over beer (as a grown man, that was a very difficult thing for me to type.)

So obviously, I'm slightly biased towards coffee. I mean, why wouldn't I sing the praises of something I drink myself? Well, as it turns out science is on my side too (and of every coffee lover on this planet.) As such, I'm going to take a more neutral approach and give you 4 solid reasons why, as a cheerleader, you can enjoy a cup of this dark nectar of the heavens, every time you hit the mat.

"It is inhumane, in my opinion, to force people who have a genuine medical need for coffee to wait in line behind people who apparently view it as some kind of recreational activity."

– Dave Barry

Reason #1: Coffee Improves Vascular Health and Performance

It is no surprise that a cup of coffee contains caffeine which can give you a nice jolt when you need it. As such, coffee has been shown to increase focus, response times, power output, endurance and even motivation.

A study showed that when sleep-deprived trainees took caffeine before their workout, they worked just as hard as those that were well rested. But when they took another group of sleepy-heads and told them to train without the aid of caffeine, the results weren't so good; these subjects not only chose to lift lighter weights, but generally *chose* to do less work overall.

Next, you should know that the caffeine from coffee isn't as bad for you as the stuff you'd get from a can of RedBull™. Most people think that taking caffeine will sky-rocket your blood pressure and do bad things to your insides. That's all grossly exaggerated.

Drinking coffee does increase your blood pressure a little, but only for the short term. Once your body metabolizes the caffeine, it's all back to normal. In fact, the caffeine in coffee increases nitric oxide production in the interior surface of blood vessels, which actually *improves* the health of these vessels.

And here's something that will really **blow your mind:** One study showed that drinking coffee habitually for 8 weeks actually *lowered* overall blood pressure readings. Didn't expect *that*, now did ya? Amazing stuff, this coffee.

Reason #2: Coffee Helps Burn Fat!

As if allowing you to tumble with more power and for a longer period of time wasn't enough, how would you like to get slimmer and leaner as well?

Yup, coffee can do that.

Drinking it has been shown to increase your metabolic rate. Basically, this means that you'll burn more calories than you normally would. Also, caffeine slows glycogen depletion (the use of sugar by your muscles) by telling your body to use fat as a preferred fuel source.

And if your body is using fat instead of glycogen, it means you'll have more fuel left over for later. You know, in case you feeling like tumbling for another hour or so. Now don't go thinking that just drinking a cup of coffee during tumbling practice will magically give you a chiseled stomach; it won't.

But if you already eat decently and condition on the regular, then adding something like green coffee extract (which is *even more* effective at burning fat than regular coffee) can definitely help your stomach go from a flat to defined; a four pack to a six.

I think you get my point – it's not magic, but it can take you to the next level if you're *already* doing the right things.

Reason #3: Coffee Helps You Live Longer

It's one thing to look good, but it's another thing to look good for a long time. Well, now we can have both because an observational study of more than 400,000 people found that the more coffee people generally drank, the longer they lived.

Men who drink about 2 cups a day dropped their risk of morality by 10 percent. For women, these results were even more favorable (more time for those selfies, huh ladies?)

Some of you might think that this whole life-extending benefit of coffee only affects a select group of people, but not so. The increase in average lifespan of coffee drinkers has been proven over a variety of different ethnicities. Basically, coffee beans don't judge – they'll help you live longer no matter what your skin colour or background. Just as how things should be.

Finally, coffee has also been associated with lowering the risk of breast, stomach, colon and lung cancer. How much lower are we talking? Well obviously it differs for each body part, but generally speaking the risk is lowered anywhere from 10 to 25 percent. Obviously, these numbers aren't mind-blowing but hey, as a coffee lover, I'll take it.

Reason #4: Coffee Helps Reduce Soreness And Speeds Up Recovery

If you've ever read my blog, then in article *6 Ways To Reduce Soreness After Tumbling Practice*, I explained how something called antioxidants can help relieve pain by reducing the inflammation in your muscles, and speed up recovery.

Well, guess what is absolutely loaded with antioxidants? Yup, coffee!

However there's one small problem... after you train hard for an hour or more, your body produces something called cortisol – also known as "the stress hormone." While cortisol has its uses, prolonged levels of cortisol in your blood have been known to have negative effects such as (but not limited to):

- Increase in fat storage near the stomach
- Slower wound/injury healing
- Impaired memory
- Decreased thyroid function
- Decrease bone density

It should be obvious that you should help your body get rid of this stuff as soon as possible. However, taking caffeine after a workout not only *elevates* the level of cortisol in your body, but it will slow down your body's ability to metabolize it.

And what has caffeine in it? Yup, coffee!

So what is a coffee lover to do? Simple, after your workout have a cup of decaffeinated coffee along with 1-2 grams of Vitamin C. This way, you get all the antioxidant goodness from coffee, and none of the drawbacks of elevated cortisol. What's more, Vitamin C will actually help your body get rid of the cortisol that's already in your system *even faster*.

All this boils down to one simple fact – you'll be able to walk into the gym sooner with less soreness and pain.

Remember: Not All Coffee Is Made Equal

So clearly, we can now conclude that coffee is awesome and that as a cheerleader, you can enjoy a cup when you're in the mood. But before you go chugging down gallons of the stuff, I need to address some common sense issues so you're not bouncing off the walls 24/7, driving your parents and coaches mad.

First, when I say coffee, I mean *actual* coffee. Not the over-priced crap you get from Starbies which is basically milk and diabetes in a cup. A Caramel Frappuccino is not going to help you recover or provide the benefits I've listed in the past few pages. I'm talking about a cup of the good ol' dark stuff with a couple shots of cream and maybe two sugars. For my Canadian friends, a double-double is the perfect choice.

If you prefer to brew your own coffee at home, I recommend buying **organic coffee** beans, as the quality and aroma are not only superior, but their antioxidant levels are much higher.

More info: http://thecheerdiet.com/links/coffee

Curcumin

As an athlete, I'm sure you're no stranger to injuries – bumps, scrapes, aches and pains are all part of the game. Obviously, you can reduce your chances of getting injured by training smart, doing a proper warm up, keeping your body strong and well-conditioned etc., but in a sport that has so much going on, things are bound to go wrong at some point.

Take a sprained ankle for example – assuming you didn't break anything major, what is the most common prescription you most likely get from a doctor?

Rest, ice and an Advil™. I can't tell you how many times athletes complain about spending hours in a waiting room to see a doctor, only to be told to rest it, wrap it and then take a pill for the pain.

Personally, I stay away from medication unless it's a last resort. In fact, I can't remember taking any type of pain medication in the past 5 years – and I've suffered lower back injuries, thumb dislocations, shoulder sprains, quad tears and a whole bunch of other bumps along the way. And I've never had to stay away from the gym for more than a week at most.

How? Well curcumin definitely gets a big chunk of the credit. So before you take some, what exactly is it?

It's a compound found in turmeric and has a yellow pigment. Turmeric as you may or may not know, is the key ingredient in curry – and curcumin is how it gets its distinctive color. But this isn't about eating curry (although it *is* rather delicious). What we're interested in, is the curcuminoid molecule that has shown to have a whole bunch of awesome benefits, two of which that are of great interest to us:

1. Powerful anti-inflammatory
2. Powerful pain reliever

Now first, you should know that inflammation is not inherently bad. It is a mechanism that our body uses to fight off bacteria, nasty pathogens and other viruses that would otherwise kill us. It also has a role in helping you heal – that's why when you sprain an ankle, it swells up.

But that's short term inflammation. What you want to avoid is any long term inflammation. Why? Because it has been shown to be a factor in many major diseases [13,14].

To help with this, there are drugs out there that can help manage inflammation, but why bother? Studies have proven that Curcumin can be just as effective as these drugs[15] and on top of that, it has a very high safety limit[16]. As in, it's very hard for you to take too much and suffer side effects – though I wouldn't recommend you pushing the limits on such things.

As for pain relief, well that goes hand-in-hand with the point I made above; as inflammation goes down, so will the pain.

Recommended Dose: First you need to decide when to take it. There are two ways to go about this – if you're old enough (18+) then taking it daily is not a bad option since it has other benefits such as boosting brain function[17], increasing mood by acting as an anti-depressant[18], helping fight off Alzheimer's and helping prevent cancer. If you are under parental supervision (or if you're a parent reading this) and have recent injuries that you need to deal with, then taking it for the duration of your healing process is a good idea. The one problem with curcumin is that your body is terrible at absorbing it, and so it needs a little assistance. There's a compound known as piperine (basically, black pepper) which can increase the absorption by 2000%. The commercial brand name for it is Bioperine[TM]. My advice would be anywhere from 300-500 mg/day with added Bioperine so be sure to look for that on the bottle.

Here's one I'd recommend:
http://thecheerdiet.com/links/curcumin

Coconut Oil & Water

As you very well know, coconut oil is chock full of benefits – but the love for coconut oil didn't always exist. In fact, as far as public image is concerned, coconut oil had a rough past and has only recently recovered its tarnished reputation.

So what went wrong?

Well there were studies which showed that coconut oil clogged arteries, raised bad cholesterol (LDL) and would increase one's risk of heart attacks. And you know what? These conclusions weren't incorrect – after all, data never lies.

But the dorky scientists conveniently forgot to mention that the *type* of coconut oil they used during their studies went through a process called hydrogenation – which produces is trans-fats. And trans-fat is some very nasty stuff. It's so bad, that New York City has actually banned[21] all restaurants from putting it in their food, and the FDA is planning on banning it altogether in the United States[22].

It turns out when you use **virgin coconut oil**, virtually everything that was a negative turns into a positive – yet more proof that trying to perfect Mother Nature is a fool's errand. I'd recommend using it anytime you do any cooking.

As it's not just the oil of coconuts that is beneficial, it turns out **coconut water** is some pretty amazing stuff too. I call it nature's sports drink because it contains the five essential electrolytes which our bodies need when we push it to the limit: magnesium, calcium, phosphorous, potassium and sodium. It's probably the ideal drink to consume *during* training because it's easier to consume in larger quantities and is quite low in calories.

Here's what one study[23] had to say:

"CW (coconut water) was significantly sweeter, caused less nausea, fullness and no stomach upset and was also easier to consume in a larger amount compared with CEB (carb-electrolyte beverage) and PW (plain water) ingestion. In conclusion, ingestion of fresh young coconut water, a natural refreshing beverage, could be used for whole body rehydration after exercise."

What's more, if you've ever suffered from muscle cramps in the past, then chances are it's because your potassium levels were too low. Fortunately, potassium levels in coconut water are well over ten times the amount you'll find in Gatorade™ or any other leading sports drink. Heck, it even has more than a banana. But since it's a liquid, your body will absorb it quicker.

My recommendation is to buy coconut water in its purest form. This means no added sugars, preservatives, colors etc. You can usually get a can of the stuff for a fairly reasonable price and drink it when you're about 30 to 40 minutes into your training session.

Why wait that long? Because while coconut water is low in calories, it's not calorie free. It also contains a bit of sugar. But if you've been following the protocols of *The Cheer Diet* correctly, then your pre-training meal is already providing you with the energy you need; your muscles already have glucose available to them. What the coconut water will do is give you that pick-me-up when you start to sweat profusely, and begin feeling a dip in your energy levels.

Finally, it bares mentioning that coconut water is **not** a complete substitute for regular water. Regardless of how long you or intense your training session is, if you timed your pre-training meal properly, one can of coconut water is all you'll need. After that, just rehydrate with water. This pre-training meal and coconut water combo is the one-two punch to having never ending energy during practices while avoiding cramps and other uncomfortable situations. You should never need to buy another bottle of Gatorade™ ever again.

The Student-Friendly Grocery List

As if the awesome information on the food pyramid wasn't enough, I'm about to give you a gift that'll keep on giving for the next 5 to 10 years of your life (assuming you plan on going to college, which I hope you do).

So what is it? It's a well thought out grocery list that is easy on the wallet, high in quality and simple to follow. You see, I've already been through the roller coaster of a ride that is high school and college, and what you're about to read is the information I *wish* I had access to.

Believe me, the "freshman 15" is very real – and what it does to people is not pretty. You don't have to live off TV dinners, cans of RedBull and pizza pockets to get you by. There is a better way that'll work out cheaper in the long run. Below are a list of foods that you can stick to, and completely live off of:

Item #1: Meat (Chicken, Lean Beef or Pork)

I love a good T-Bone steak just like anyone else (well, except vegetarians, of course) but having it constantly can make you poor rather quickly. Instead, these are the 3 types of meats which go on sale *very* often. And when they do, be sure to buy a crap load and throw it in the freezer.

Now depending on where you live, you'll have to know what constitutes as a "good" price. If you've never done your own grocery shopping before, I suggest you start now because it's a very useful life skill. For those in North America, look for prices that are around **$2.99/pound or less**. As soon as you see this, snatch it up!

A good trick you can use for ground beef is to look for stuff that's *not* too lean. The price difference between beef that's 85% lean vs 95% is significant (usually by a few dollars per pound!) So get the 85. As you know by now, the extra fat isn't going to do any harm.

For chicken, buying breasts that come with skin will also save you a significant amount of cash. And the best part? You can cook your chicken with the skin as it helps it stay moist and juicy. You only have to remove it right before you eat it. Sounds like a win – win to me.

Item #2: Eggs (whole)

One of the guys I've studied and looked up to over the years is Charles Poliquin – he's arguably one of the most accomplished and successful strength coaches in the world. He's helped more Olympians achieve podium results than I can recall. Needless to say when he talks, I listen. One of his famous quotes is *"Egg whites are for dorks!"*

I couldn't agree more. Removing the most nutritious part of the egg and throwing it away is an absolute crime. Not only does the yolk contain half the protein, but it also contains HDL (if you remember, that's the *good* cholesterol). So eat the damn yolk! The great news is that eggs are not only cheap, but very easy to make (as you'll soon see in the recipe section). Usually, 15 minutes is all you need to make any competent egg dish. When it comes to pricing, eggs vary quite a bit; in the US I've heard you can get a **dozen for $2**, which to me is nuts, so if you can approach that price anywhere, stock up!

Item #3: Tuna

I know, this should be listed with the other meats, but I felt it was important enough to get its own section since it's so convenient - you can eat it right out of the can! The great thing about tuna is that every week, there is always some type of brand that's on sale. Look for prices that approach **a dollar per can**. Now I get it - eating non-prepared tuna might not be the most delicious option, but trust me, when you're in a pinch, getting your protein after a hard practice is much more important than satisfying your taste buds. Also note, other types of canned fish such as salmon, sardines and tilapia can also go on sale and make for a great alternative. Shop around!

Item #4: Oatmeal

A great source of LG carbs, provided you don't ruin it by drowning it in sugar. Now for the purposes of this cost-conscious list, I'm not talking about the flavored packets of oatmeal, though if you have the extra cash you can certainly enjoy those once in a while.

What I've listed here is the plain, regular oatmeal that you can customize how you like. You know what I'm talking about – the big 5 pound bag of the stuff. Personally, I like putting bananas in mine and pairing it with a cup of coffee. Usually, you should get about 30 grams of quality carbs per serving, and if you get it at a low enough price (**say $3 or less**) then you could end up paying only $0.1 per serving. That's absolutely *insane!*

Item #5: Powdered Milk

I call this the poor man's protein powder because while whey is absolutely awesome, it's not cheap if you want to get the right stuff. During my college years, this was one of the best "hacks" that I came across which allowed me to keep my protein intake up. Not only is it almost as good as regular milk, but get it on sale and you can literally cut your milk spending in **half!** All while getting the benefits of protein, vitamin D and calcium.

And because it's powdered, *you* control the consistency. So if you like milkshakes, this is a great option. Oh and if you can get your hands on cheap chocolate syrup, it's game over! You'll instantly get access to the best tasting and the most inexpensive pre and post workout drink on Earth.

Item #6: Greek Yogurt

Delicious, convenient, high in protein, and relatively inexpensive – what's not to love about this stuff? I usually don't like to buy fat free *anything*, but in terms of Greek yogurt, 0% tends to have higher amounts of protein. But 2% is still a great option; goes well with almonds!

Item #7: Beans & Lentils

I think beans get an unfair reputation as being nothing more than ammo to produce ear-shattering farts. But that's not always true. The great thing about beans is that they're not only inexpensive, but they're an excellent source of quality fibre and protein, which means they can help you feel fuller for longer. Another plus is that they're usually low glycemic – which means no crazy spikes in blood sugar, giving you a stable stream of energy for hours. Sounds good right? But wait, there's more!

There was a study[19] which found that those who frequently consumed beans in their diet were 22% less likely to be obese, 23% less likely to have a fat gut, and had lower blood pressure when compared to those that didn't eat beans at all. This is a significant boost! As if that wasn't enough, it turns out that being a female bean consumer can have an even bigger upside; a review which looked at the diet and nutrition data of about 90,000 women discovered the following:

*"scientists at the Harvard School of Public Health found that those who ate beans and lentils at least twice a week **had a 25 percent lower risk of breast cancer** than women who ate them just once a month."*[20]

Those are some impressive benefits for a food group that's so easy on the wallet and totally delicious when cooked right. What's more, when you compare real world, practical observation to these studies, the results are in complete alignment. Here's what I mean:

Dan Buettner is a man who set out to find the specific places on Earth where people are consistently living the longest (around 100 years) and to see if there were any commonalities in their lifestyles, and if so, how we could benefit off of their practical, tried-and-true wisdom.

And find these places he did!

Dan calls them BlueZones, and wrote an entire book about it (which I highly recommend you read). But for now I'll give you the basic gist of things. Here are the Bluezones that Dan found:

- Okinawa, Japan
- Ikaria, Greece
- Sardinia, Italy
- Nicoya, Costa Rica
- Loma Linda, California

Inside these five Bluezones, Dan found that there were 9 specific things they were doing, which resulted in the population enjoying a long, healthy and prosperous life. And can you guess what one of those 9 things were?

Yup, the consumption of beans and lentils!

(Also here's a fun side-note for all the parents and coaches reading this: The populations from 4 out of the 5 Bluezones consumed alcohol regularly – so go ahead, enjoy your wine)

Now I'm not here to conclude that by simply consuming beans (or wine), you'll magically live to be a 100. But if some of the world's healthiest, and longest living people are eating it on a regular basis, we should pay attention and seriously consider including it in our diet.

So what type of beans should you get? I'd say aim to get white and black beans, as their protein content is some of the highest*. Beans can be used to make awesome companion dishes to meats, and you can also use them to make chili – one of my personal favorite foods.

*Highest next to soybeans – which I would avoid as they are some of the most genetically modified food products out there, and are sprayed with a ridiculous amount of pesticide. My stance on GMO's is the same as aspartame – avoiding it results in a net positive. So why take the chance?

Item #8: Home Made Frozen Vegetables

You know you need to eat your veggies, but here's the major problem – veggies can go bad very quickly, and if you're busy then you can't keep buying tiny amounts of the stuff every time you need to prepare a meal or salad. You could buy frozen, but that comes at a cost.

The solution? Spend half an hour once every two weeks making your own frozen vegetables! Here's the basic, 3 step process:

Step 1: Buy and prep your vegetables. I don't care which ones you get – a good rule of thumb is to cover all the colors of the veggie spectrum (white, green, red, yellow, orange, purple). If you do this, you'll be well off. Then just wash and chop them up into sizes that you prefer. Use a good, sharp knife and make sure you're under parental supervision.

Step 2: Prepare a large pot by filling it with water and bringing it to a boil. Also, have another pot on the side filled with ice cold water. Now we do something called blanching – place your chopped up veggies inside the boiling pot of water for about 3 minutes. Once the time is up, toss them in the ice cold water for 5-10 seconds then drain and pat dry with a paper towel.

Step 3: Place your blanched veggies on a baking tray and freeze until they're rock hard. Then just place them inside zip lock bags and store in the freezer for future use.

If you're OCD then you can blanche each color on its own. But if you're lazy like me, just mix it all together. The great thing is that these frozen veggies can be taken from the freezer to the plate and microwaved for about 2-3 minutes for instant consumption. You can literally make a boat load of frozen veggies in about half an hour and for about half the price you would normally have to pay.

Chapter 4: Putting It All Together, And Starting Your 60 Day Plan

Get Your Mind Right

At this point, you may feel overwhelmed with all the information you've just read. And I don't blame you - it's a lot to take in, especially if you've never had a "behind the scenes" access on something you thought was so simple – eating food.

But don't worry, implementing *The Cheer Diet* is actually not hard at all. I've broken the 60 day process into three distinct phases, and all you have to do is follow them in order.

You should mentally prepare yourself to **treat the diet like any other skill.** For example, you don't learn a layout full twist before learning the round off, back handspring, back tuck, back pike, layout etc., and mastering this diet works similarly. Think of each phase as a progression that's designed to help your body adapt to specific areas of performance eating.

Also, should you have minor setbacks, don't let these small failures define who you are, or what you're capable of. For example: when a flyer becomes loose and falls out of a stunt that she's been able to hit before, does that mean she's now a terrible athlete?

Heck no.

Or say a cheerleader is trying to learn a front tuck, and after weeks of doing drills and getting spotted, her first attempt results in a hilarious butt stomp. Does this mean she's doomed, and not meant to tumble? Of course not, that would be a ridiculous conclusion! If she wants it, she'll get up, fix what went wrong, and try again.

So if you happen to slip during this 60 day process, or your willpower doesn't hold up, just go all Taylor Swift on it and *"shake it off."* Then continue onwards! Accidentally eating a cookie on a day you're not supposed to won't throw off the whole thing, so make sure the rest of your week doesn't suffer due to one small slip. Learn from it, fix it, and carry on.

The Structure Of The Diet

The underlying structure (or the core philosophy) of *The Cheer Diet* is as simple and logical as it gets: **on days you train, eat more, on days you don't, eat less.**

Based on what you've read in the previous chapters, the reason behind this structure should be glaringly obvious: when you train, your body obviously needs fuel, so you should be eating more. However on days you don't train, the body only needs enough to stay alive and recover. Therefore eating more will only result in fat being stored in places which you don't want.

Before we dive into each one of the phases, I should remind you to complete the 7 Day Habit Cue Log. It isn't part of the 60 day plan per say, but as you know from Chapter 2, it's still a very important piece of the puzzle. You need to log and understand your behavior so that you can work with your body instead of against it. This will help conserve willpower for the important stuff.

Phase 1: Calorie Reset (14 Days)

If you remember from my version of the food pyramid, the amount of calories is the most important factor of any diet. So the goal of the first phase is to train your body (specifically, the gut bacteria levels in your stomach and your hunger signals) to adapt and get used to eating just the right amount of calories, regardless of your current eating habits (however great or poor they may be).

So if you're a chronic over-eater, this phase will help you eat less. If you're an under-eater then you'll now be eating the amount of food you *should* have been eating all along.

Naturally, the question that's probably on your mind is, *"So how do I know how many calories to eat?"*

Well, I promised you that counting calories is not something you're going to have to worry about on *The Cheer Diet*, so for phase one there are 3 simple rules you'll follow:

1. **Eat only 3 meals per day & time them with your cues**
2. **No fast food, junk food or snacking allowed**
3. **You must cook/prepare your meals**

Ideally, I'd recommend going into the recipe section and picking the meals from there (obviously the smoothies are off limits during phase one). If you want to be ideal, pick 2 low carb meals and one high carb. Also, know that taking seconds or going over the portion limits set in the recipe section is not allowed. Aim to eat exactly what the recipe defines as a portion, and save the rest for later.

Phase 1 FAQ

Q: What do I do for school? I can prepare my breakfast but for lunch, I usually buy food.

Then you need to prepare in advance. The secondary reason for phase one is to teach you how to take charge of your own nutrition and eating habits – and this means not relying on mommy to do everything for you. Buy some Tupperware containers, cook your meals on the weekend and store them in the fridge. The meals will last a week and all you'll need to do is reheat them. Most school kitchens should allow you to re-heat your food. However, if your school serves a healthy lunch and you really cannot prep in advance then go ahead and get something – but remember, no seconds.

Q: I snack constantly throughout the day. What do I do if I feel hungry during this phase?

Let's talk about hunger real quick. The first thing you need to remember about hunger, is that 99% of the time (especially in today's world), it is *not* a survival response. What I mean by this, is that your body doesn't give you hunger pangs because it needs calories to stay alive, it gives them to you based on **habit**.

So when you feel hungry, first remind yourself that you're just fine, that the feeling is temporary. And don't forget the research we talked about earlier – it takes 3 days of *total fasting* for your body's metabolism to drop, so it's not like you're going to die because you skipped a few snacks.

I know hunger is an uncomfortable feeling, so the best solution is to drink a big glass of water. Also remember, you have science on your side when it comes to the rules of this phase – eating 3 big meals with protein in it is far superior for appetite control, so you really shouldn't feel too hungry if you follow the recipes I've laid out.

Q: I usually don't eat this much food, and feel unusually full during my days. Is this normal?

Yup. As an under-eater, you will have the exact opposite problem as the over-eaters did in the question above. Since your body is not used to having so much food come in, it needs time to adapt. This is why phase one lasts 14 days. By the end of these two weeks, both groups of athletes (under-eaters and over-eaters) should have adapted just fine, and any odd fullness feelings or hunger pangs should go away completely, if not mostly. My sneaky tip for under-eaters is to eat quickly, as it takes the brain anywhere from 10-20 minutes to realize you're full and fire off the "fullness" feeling you get.

Q: I'm very OCD and don't mind counting calories – in fact I'd like to know how much to eat daily. Can you tell me?

If you're hell-bent on making things more complicated for yourself, then sure, take your bodyweight in pounds and multiply that number by 12.5 – that's how many daily calories you'll need to aim for during phase one.

Q: What about training and meal timing? Should I worry about this as explained in the pyramid?

Yup, you still want to make sure you're not eating your meals too close to your training sessions – this is one of those times where you'll have to go against your habit cues. So for example, if you know you always eat *right* before you leave for practice, you'll need to beat this cue by an hour or two to reprogram your habit. More on meal timing will be explained in the next phase. Having said that, timing your meals perfectly is *not* the priority of phase one, so if you feel like it's robbing too much of your willpower, just worry about the three rules outlined above.

Phase 2: Alternating Meal Planning (14 days)

If you truly stuck to your cues and completed phase one, then go ahead and take a cheat day to celebrate (this day doesn't count towards the 60). If there were any snacks that you were craving, the cheat day will allow you to enjoy them – but please use common sense. For example, if you missed cheesecake dearly then have a small slice instead of the entire cake.

The goal of phase 2 is to introduce you (and your body) to taking in **training-specific** amount of calories. Phase one evened out the rough edges by forcing those who eat too much to eat less, and those who ate too little, to eat more. So now, you're ready to eat like a true athlete and allow your body to be in fat burning mode when needed, and to really provide you with energy during practices. The rules for Phase 2 are as follows:

1. **On training days, eat any 3 meals**
2. **On rest days, eat 2 low carb meals + 1 smoothie**
3. **No junk/fast food or random snacking allowed**

A few details I should point out: The 3 meals on training days can now be almost anything you like – but just like in phase one, extra servings aren't allowed.

I also recommend you eat lots of quality carbs (things like sweet potatoes, oatmeal, brown rice etc.) But if you want to make one of the meals into something convenience oriented such as a protein shake or a smoothie, then feel free to do that as well. I should really call it 3 eating "sessions," but you get the idea.

For rest days, the low carb meals should come from the recipe section – as they've been specifically designed with the correct portions and ingredients for athletes. Also, if you want to see examples then don't worry, after the 3 phases are explained I'll show you what an ideal week would look like. You can then use these examples as a model.

Phase 3: The Cheer Diet (32 days)

This is it young lady, the very diet this *entire* book is based on. As you'll soon see based on the rules, there's a very good reason the first 2 phases were needed - because jumping into this phase cold-turkey can be a bit overwhelming for your body (though I'd be lying if I said it *can't* be done).

In this full-fledged plan, each day (training or rest) has its own set of rules so I suggest writing them down somewhere for easy reference. But don't worry, after eating the way of *The Cheer Diet* for the next 32 days, it will become second nature – you'll naturally start to make the right choices and have awesome practices to boot! Let's jump right in.

Training Day Rules

1. **Eat 2 high carb meals** (either based on old cues or pick different ones if you want to build a new habit)
2. **Consume a smoothie 45-60 minutes before practice** (or take in one serving of HG carbs*)
3. **After practice consume one of the following:** protein smoothie, a general protein shake or a low carb meal.

Rest Day Rules

1.   **Eat any 2 low carb meals of your choice**
2.   **Have any one smoothie of your choice**
3.   **Avoid HG carbs and junk food at *all costs!***

Global Rules

- Track your measurements weekly (stick into BF Calculator)
- Add a cheat day after every 2 weeks on Phase 3

** If for some reason you can't manage to make a pre-workout smoothie during training days, try and prepare it in advance and toss it in a cooler. If that's not possible, you may have some High Glycemic carbs to fuel your training session as long as you take it within 45 - 60 mins **before** training. Below is a list of HG carbs I've successfully used in the past for a quick boost (remember, you **shouldn't have more than one serving**, which is about a handful).*

- *Low fiber fruits*
- *Muffins*
- *Nutella (you may use the sandwich recipe listed in chapter 6)*
- *Chocolate Bars (if you're under 5 feet tall, you may only have **half the serving**. So for example if you picked up a KitKat bar, eat only 2 of the fingers. My favorite chocolate bars of all time: KitKat, Twix, Snickers, OhHenry, EatMore, Wunderbar, Crunch)*
- *Cereal with milk (My personal favorites: Cinnamon Toast Crunch or Coco Puffs)*
- *Donuts/Pastries*

Lastly, don't forget that your body needs water to absorb carbohydrates, so drink a full glass of water after taking in your HG carbs, and keep sipping throughout your practice.

More Details On Tracking Your Progress

Here's a quote I constantly refer to with my clients and athletes: *"You cannot improve what you don't measure."* And it's true – how do you know something is working, unless you have hard data to back it up? You might think that by having more energy during practices, fitting better in your clothes and getting compliments are all signs of progress. And that's true, but those don't come during the first week.

When someone loses half an inch off their waist, that's a sign of progress, but would they be able to tell by looking in the mirror? Probably not.

Yet knowing this piece of information can be crucial – it can let us know if the plan is working, or if adjustments need to be made. I mean, who wants to put in a month's worth of work only to realize that 10 days into the plan, the diet should've been tweaked? No one.

That's why I like to measure the smallest details every week so that I know I'm on the right path – even if it doesn't feel like so. As you'll recall, *The Cheer Diet* isn't concerned with weight. I know it's nice to see a drop in the scale (which young lady wouldn't want that?) but you have to remember, we're after a body that helps you become a better *athlete*. This means outright weight is irrelevant.

So what *should* we be measuring?

The answer is your body fat levels (the ratio between how much muscle you have vs body fat). Here's something that'll blow your mind: I've had powerlifters that came to me for nutrition planning and after 6 months, their weight remained almost completely unchanged.

Now on the surface this sounds terrible: *"six months and they didn't even lose a pound?!"*

But if you were to look at them, the difference was night and day. Their "after" picture contained abs, muscle definition in their legs and arms, and more energy than they knew what to do with.

In other words, they got "toned." So what's the easiest way to know you're on a one-way trip to ToneVille?

To track your body fat percentage – and it's not as hard as it sounds. In fact, I've made it dead simple. All you'll need to do is get the following measurements: height, neck, waist and hips. Then stick those numbers into the convenient Excel calculator that I've created, and it will spit out the Bodyfat % for you. From there all you need to do is make sure that percentage is dropping from week-to-week by keeping an eye on the included graph, simple! You'll definitely need an accurate tape measure for this, so be sure to buy one.

How To Work The Excel BodyFat Calculator

To get access to the calculator, head over to the resource page (http://bit.ly/cheerfiles - password: **tcd2015**) and download it. Upon opening, you'll see a picture that shows you exactly how to take the measurements. Then it's just a matter of sticking the numbers into the yellow boxes and placing the result into the weekly progress chart.

The calculator comes filled with "dummy data" so you can get an idea of how it works. Play around with it and have some fun.

Note: the body fat calculator works with inches by default, but if you work better with the Metric system, then you're out of luck! Just kidding – all you have to do is take your metric measurements, and stick them into the included converter before plugging in your numbers. You didn't *really* think I'd leave you hanging now did you?

Phase 3 FAQ

Q: Should I be tracking my BodyFat % in the first 2 phases?

Absolutely not. The goal of the first 2 phases is adaption. Now this doesn't mean you won't see progress during the first 2 phases, but I don't want you to get stressed out about it. You won't experience all the benefits of *The Cheer Diet* till phase 3, so that's when you should start to measure progress.

Q: What about supplements like multivitamins and such?

You should be taking your multi everyday regardless of the phase. As far as the other supplements go, use as directed and for the right reasons. If you're unsure, be sure to talk with your doctor.

Q: Do the meals have to come from the included recipes?

While I do recommend you follow the included recipes as often as possible, in phase 3 it is assumed that you know and have enough experience to explore your boundaries without violating the rules of the diet. As an example, if you don't feel like cooking or you're out at dinner on your rest day, then ditching the fries with your burger for a salad is a pretty smart idea since veggies with high water content (such as lettuce) don't contain too many carbs or calories. The burger on the other hand, is likely high in protein and the total carbs from the bun will likely keep you within your daily limits. Or to play it really safe, you can ditch the bun and just have the burger patty with your salad and a glass of juice. See? Simple.

Q: I feel like I can totally do phase 3 without going through the first two, so can I...

STOP! Don't do it. I specifically designed this whole 60 day process for a reason. A lot of thought, careful planning and testing have gone into this. Trust me, you *need* to do the phases in order. You wouldn't skip a progression when it comes to learning a cheer skill, so don't skip the phases.

Q: What do I do after Phase 3?

The final phase is infinite – as an athlete it is how you should be eating and fueling yourself. Basically, your job is to turn phase 3 into a lifestyle; a habitual pattern that sticks. And yes, the global cheat day rule still applies; once every 2 weeks you may take a day where you go absolutely bananas and eat whatever your heart desires. Enjoy! ☺

Q: Can I have a cheat day once a week instead?

Not a chance.

Nice try though.

Phase 1 Example Log

Since phase 1 is straight forward, I created a log that spans three days so you can get a glimpse of what an ideal situation would look like. The high carb/high calorie meals are listed in bold. Also note that I've created this log using lots of meal options – this is great if you get bored easily and want to keep your taste buds excited. However, I will say that a more consistent approach is not only more manageable, but is cheaper while grocery shopping since you're not forced to buy 20 different ingredients.

Day	Recipes Used
Mon	Vegetable Omelette Meat Rollups **Spicy Beef Chili**
Tue	Coach Sahil's Scrambled Eggs Beef Kebabs **Tuna Pizza w/ Chocolate Milk**
Wed	Strawberries w/ Greek Yogurt Easy Chicken & Rice **Nutella & Banana Sandwich**

Phase 2 Example Log

Recall the rules for phase 2 are as follows: **On training days, eat any 3 meals. On rest days, eat 2 low carb meals + 1 smoothie. No junk/fast food or random snacking allowed.** The "T" stands for training day.

Day	Recipes Used
Mon (T) RPE: 7	Steak & Veggie Stir Fry Vanilla Spice Blueberry Oatmeal Salad
Tue	Vegetable Omelette Easy Chicken & Rice Smoothie #6
Wed (T) RPE: 8	Strawberries w/ Greek Yogurt Steak & Veggie Stir Fry Vanilla Spice Blueberry Oatmeal
Thurs	Vegetable Omelette Easy Chicken & Rice Smoothie #4
Fri (T) REP: 8	Scrambled Eggs Steak & Veggie Stir Fry Vanilla Spice Blueberry Oatmeal
Sat	Beef Kebabs Easy Chicken & Rice Smoothie #2
Sun	Mushroom Omelette Easy Chicken & Rice Smoothie #4

Notice how I've kept the training day meals and the rest day meals relatively consistent. For example, chicken and rice is almost a staple on this person's rest day plan whereas during training days, one of the meals is always oatmeal – to provide energy during practices. The timing of these meals will obviously differ based on when you train and your habitual patterns. Finally, you'll notice the words "RPE" - what do they mean, and why is the Monday training session a 7? You'll learn more about that in chapter seven.

Phase 3 Example Log

To keep things simple, I've carried over the same training schedule from the phase 2 example log, and adjusted the recipes to fit the rules of phase 3. You may follow this exact plan, or play around and come up with your own.

Day	Recipes Used
Mon (T) RPE: 7	Vanilla Spice Blueberry Oatmeal Spicy Beef Chili Smoothie #3 Protein Shake
Tue	Vegetable Omelette Easy Chicken & Rice Smoothie #6
Wed (T) RPE: 8	Steak & Veggie Stir Fry Chocolate Banana Oatmeal Smoothie #8 Smoothie #8 w/ whey protein
Thurs	Coach Sahil's Scrambled Eggs Easy Chicken & Rice Smoothie #4
Fri (T) REP: 8	Chicken Nuggets w/ Squash Chocolate Banana Oatmeal Smoothie #8 Meal Rollups
Sat	Beef Kebabs Easy Chicken & Rice Smoothie #2
Sun	Mushroom Omelette Easy Chicken & Rice Smoothie #4

Chapter 5: Handling The "Lady Factors" That Might Affect The Diet

I know it's not exactly a hot topic to discuss, but I figured if this book was to be the *complete* nutrition guide for female cheerleaders, I'd have to talk about the "p" word at some point.

And no, I'm not referring to **ponies.**

So why discuss it? Because the simple fact of the matter is, 75% of women aged 18 and over suffer from some type of premenstrual discomfort, and for 20% out of those women, the discomfort is so severe, that they usually need some type of medical assistance; these include prescription medications such as danazol - a drug that suppresses ovulation and causes increased facial hair and acne.

Newer drugs called gonadatropin-releasing hormone (GnRH) actually change brain chemistry to turn off the ovaries' production of estrogen and progesterone, which sounds great — but they can also lead to osteoporosis. Other times, diuretics are used to treat fluid retention. (A diuretic is a substance that promotes the production of urine. Basically, it helps the body pee out its fluid stores, which can be useful but only at very specific times.)

Now, I've handled diet plans for plenty of women in the past, and have found that adopting a healthier lifestyle can have a dramatic impact on their PMS symptoms. In fact, special adjustments to the diet don't usually need to be made.

Having said that, I'm still going to take things a step further, and show you how to optimize *The Cheer Diet* so you can get the upper hand on Mother Nature, should you be one of the unlucky ones. Before we go any further, the *very* first thing you should do is talk to your doctor (if you haven't already) to find out whether or not you actually suffer from PMS.

If you don't currently have a family doctor, I'd get a couple of opinions (both from male and female doctors) just to be sure, because it's seriously easier to diagnose the flu than it is PMS. The reason for this is that the symptom list is huge and it can be tricky, even for doctors, to be absolutely sure about a PMS diagnosis when they aren't familiar with your medical history. As an example, below is a brief list of these symptoms:

- Hot flashes
- Weight gain
- Severe headaches
- Sudden depression or sadness
- Bloating
- Fatigue
- Cramps
- Anti-Social behaviour
- Nightmares
- Anxiety from trivial situations
- Mood swings
- Nausea
- ...and many more.

Again, that's not all the symptoms because if I were to list them all, it'd probably fill two entire pages. But the general consensus is that if you suffer from five or more of the ones listed above, there's a very good chance that you suffer from PMS (again, check with your doctor to be sure!)

Now, if you're one of the lucky ones who only has to deal with minor inconveniences for a day or two, then you may skip this chapter entirely. But if you're someone who turns into Regina George with the temper of Eddie Rios*, then just know that through quality nutrition you can dramatically decrease your level of discomfort.

Let's start with a list of things you should avoid...

Stress or Stressful Situations

It might seem obvious, but you'll really have to make a conscious effort to eject yourself from the vicinity of people who know how to push your buttons. You may generally be a calm and positive person, but we both know how short your fuse can get during these times. What's more, stress drives up cortisol, and cortisol can increase your levels of belly fat, and that's the last thing you want.

Carbonated Beverages

While this isn't allowed on *The Cheer Diet* anyways, I had to give it a special mention because being in a lousy or cranky mood can drive your sugar cravings up the wall, and you may want to reach for a can of pop. But don't! The carbonation can cause some serious bloating, or make it worse if you already suffer from it. Plain water or tea only is the way to go. In fact, I'll tell you the exact type of tea to drink in a moment.

"Wait coach, what about coffee? You spent a few pages recommending the stuff"

Good question, which brings us to the next substance you should avoid during this time of the month...

Caffeine

While I do indeed stand behind the merits of coffee and believe that for athletes, caffeine in *reasonable dosages* can be beneficial, you should really avoid it during these times as it can increase mood swings, anxiety, and cortisol levels. It might initially make you feel good, but you will crash, and here's why:

A 3 Minute Crash Course On How Caffeine Works

For a drug to have an effect on you, it needs to cross the BBB (blood brain barrier). Basically, think of your brain as an island surrounded by a sea of... uh, blood (bear with me on this).

And only certain ships are able to sail across. In fact, pharmaceutical companies spend a lot of money developing therapies where their drugs can cross the BBB.

Why?

Because if their drugs cannot reach the brain, those pills will be about as useful as cheap Halloween candy. Thankfully, because caffeine is both soluble in water and fat, it can cross the BBB with ease. Once inside the brain, caffeine needs to attach itself to a receptor to be effective. Receptors can be thought of as keyholes, and only specific types of keys can fit inside to unlock them.

While we don't have specific caffeine receptors, we do come loaded with adenosine receptors. And caffeine, being the sneaky substance that it is, basically impersonates adenosine and competes with it to attach to the very same receptors.

If you've ever had an energy drink in your life, then you're probably aware that caffeine usually wins this receptor battle. And when it does, it blocks the adenosine from attaching to its own receptor. Now this is where the magic happens: when adenosine is blocked from binding to its own receptor, you levels of dopamine, serotonin, noradrenaline and acetylcholine go up.

What the heck are those substances? They're neurotransmitters (if you'll remember, we talked about them from the aspartame section). Basically these specific neurotransmitters make you feel alive, alert and more focused – which is what we all love about caffeine.

But the problem is that you have a limited reserve of these neurotransmitters, and caffeine pulls in too many of them at once. It's like slamming the gas pedal on a car; the initial speed, rush and sound is exciting but it can only last so long since you're using up a massive amount of fuel every second. So when these effects wear off, the neurotransmitters levels drop like the stock market did back in 2008.

This is also known as the "caffeine crash". As if that wasn't bad enough, caffeine also blocks something called GABA (gamma aminobutyric acid) which results in anxiety, insomnia, and a rise in heartbeat. So now you're tired, moody, and for some reason your heart is pounding away like it does when you start talking to your secret crush.

And finally, let's go back to poor adenosine for a second. During the time it's being blocked from its own receptors, it obviously can't do its job – which is to be a neuroprotector. What does a neuroprotector do? It increases blood flow to the brain, down regulates brain activity and induces sleep when it feels like you're doing too much thinking for your own good.

In other words, it prevents your brain from exploding *(that may or may not be a slight exaggeration)*.

So once caffeine is done doing its thing, and the receptors are free again, all the lingering adenosine molecules *rush* back towards them, and bind to what's rightfully theirs. When this happens, they do what they're best at – protect your brain by making you feel sleepy, tired, and drowsy.

This rollercoaster of emotions piled on top of the irritability you're already going through is a recipe for turning into "that crazy chick."

Bottom Line?

Avoid caffeine during these troubled times of being a lady. A better option is tea, but not just any tea. I'll show you the specific type to drink in just a moment.

Alcohol

Not that you should be drinking this stuff anyways, but it has to be said since many countries around the world have a more favorable drinking age than Canada or the United States.

Regardless of the social situation though, I suggest saving the alcohol for when you retire from being an athlete since it's a depressant and will only bring your mood down.

Processed/High Sodium Foods

Highly processed foods are not only deprived of essential nutrients and minerals but they're also very calorie dense and take longer for your body to assimilate. This can lead to poor digestion, and it can definitely worsen PMS symptoms. How do you know your food is processed? Simple, if it came in a box, some type of pre-packaging, from fast food restaurants or has a very long shelf life, then it's most likely processed in one way or another.

While this book does have a few convenience oriented recipes based on some processed ingredients, when it comes to avoiding discomfort during PMS, stick to cooking and eating fresh ingredients as much as possible.

As for high sodium, if you avoid processed foods, you'll most likely also end up avoiding sodium (salt) as those two things go hand in hand. However, it should be said that if you're a salt lover, hold off from putting too much on your food as salt holds water, and this leads to bloating and breast tenderness during your cycle.

Sugar

Keeping your sweet tooth in check will help you avoid the peaks and valleys in your blood sugar level. When your blood sugar is stable you'll feel less fatigued. Also, too much refined (white) sugar can really rob your body of nutrients and reduce the absorption of magnesium. If you're tempted to reach for something like chocolate as a comfort food during these difficult times, reach for the dark stuff, as it actually has benefits (more on this soon).

Now that you know what to avoid, let's take a look at some foods that will actually help you...

Chamomile tea

While regular tea has less caffeine than coffee, I still suggest you try and avoid it completely. This is why Chamomile tea is awesome - it's completely caffeine free and can possibly help relieve muscle spasms, which is very good for those of you who suffer from cramps. You can think of this as the "soothing tea" as it will also help mellow out your mood. If coffee ever had an exact opposite, it would most likely be chamomile tea. Give it a try:
http://thecheerdiet.com/links/tea

Dark Chocolate

Yep, your special time of the month is actually the perfect time for some dark chocolate. I realize that I don't exactly have to provide reasons for you to follow this recommendation; telling young women to have some chocolate is like asking Miley Cyrus if she wants to come in on a wrecking ball. But for the sake of an education, here's why **dark** chocolate is awesome:

First, it just plain makes you feel good. If you read your news from an online source (highly likely) then you may have heard about the famous Harris Interactive poll[1] which circulated all over social media last year. In it, they realized that French women preferred chocolate over, ahem, more promiscuous activities. But there's definitely a reason behind it. Eating chocolate actually boosts your serotonin levels (yep, it's a neurotransmitter). Also, dark chocolate contains a decent amount of phenylethylamine – a chemical which builds up in your brain when you're in love.

So all these years, when women have claimed that they "love" chocolate, they weren't kidding!

This is all great news when you're feeling moody or down, but the benefits don't stop there. The cocoa (the base from which all chocolate is made) is one of the highest and potent sources of antioxidants.

Research shows that cocoa can do the following: "*protect nerves from injury and inflammation, protect the skin from oxidative damage from UV radiation in topical preparations, and have beneficial effects on satiety, cognitive function, and mood.*[2]"

However, because cocoa is naturally very bitter, most of it is taken out from the candy bars you buy at regular convenience stores and replaced with, you guessed it, a crap load of refined sugar and milk. Another downside is that milk can hamper with the absorption of antioxidants, so not only are you getting less, but what you are getting cannot be absorbed. This is why something like a KitKat™ isn't the best choice during your period.

Water

If eating too much sodium (salt) can cause you to hold water, and thus feel bloated, then logic tells us you should avoid drinking lots of water in the first place, right?

Wrong. Reducing your water intake, especially during your period, is definitely one of the worst things you can do because it causes your body to hang on to the fluids it already has. Drinking lots of water will help you flush things out, so drink up.

Multivitamin

Since you are losing a lot of micronutrients, you need to replace them in adequate amounts. The easiest way is to buy a regular multivitamin designed specifically for women, then double up the dosage during you period (take once in the morning and once at night). Below are some of the **micro**nutrients that offer major advantages.

Calcium: During PMS a woman's body tends to have its calcium balance out of whack, and is at an increased risk of osteoporosis. As such, one study found that getting some extra calcium in your diet can reduce your uncomfortable PMS symptoms by up to 48%! [3]

Magnesium: Not only are North Americans already deficient in this important mineral, but taking it during this time of the month can help since it improves mood and eases the irritability that you may feel. Be sure that your multi has magnesium citrate and not oxide, as its better absorbed by the body. You can also buy this stuff as standalone without breaking the bank – it's pretty inexpensive.

Vitamin D: If you live where the sun shines all year round and you're generally an outdoorsy person, then you won't have to worry about this, but for those that live in countries or areas where the seasons change dramatically, getting in at least 2000IU (international units) of Vitamin D per day for an athlete is essential.

Iron: For blood to carry adequate amounts of oxygen, it needs hemoglobin. Therefore getting enough iron is paramount, especially for a young female athlete. However, you don't need to take it constantly; a study[4] published in the *Asia Pacific Journal Of Clinical Nutrition* came to the following conclusion:

"...Weekly supplementation of iron tablets continued for 16 weeks contributed a higher improvement to hemoglobin concentration, compared with supplementing iron tablets for four consecutive days during menstruation for four menstrual cycles. This suggests that weekly iron supplementation is preferable."

Basically, once a week is more than enough, especially if you can get accustomed to eating organ meats - which are already rich in iron.

Exercise

The last thing you want to do is become a couch potato. If you follow the recommendations above, you should be able to get yourself to cheer practice without any issue. However, if you're in the off season or for whatever reason don't have any practices coming up, take time out of your day to do a workout – anything that makes you sweat will do.

The reason? It helps your body rid of excess water, and working out releases endorphins – basically natural morphine produced by your nervous system that can reduce pain felt by cramps, improve sleep, and generally uplift your mood.

Conclusion

I hope you learnt a thing or two about what your body goes through during this time of the month, and why you need to pay extra attention and take care of yourself.

Technically, just the basics of *The Cheer Diet* should help ease any irritability symptoms since you'll be eating better and providing the body with the nutrients it needs, but the special recommendations in this chapter should help you really take control of any symptoms that make you uncomfortable.

Finally, don't forget to talk with your doctor to see if they make any recommendations that are in-line with what I've listed here. In fact, I suggest going over this chapter with them since they have access to your medical history, and can give you the most accurate advice.

Chapter 6: Recipes To Use For *The Cheer Diet*

The recipe section is divided into three categories: **Low carb/Low calorie** meals (used for rest days), **High carb/High calorie** meals (used for training days), and **Smoothies.**

Once you've gone through the 60 day process, feel free to adjust, modify and play around with the recipe as you please – but make sure the numbers don't deviate too much. For example, if a low carb meal has 30g of carbs, but your variation has 60g, then that's not exactly a low carb meal anymore, is it? Common sense is your friend.

Also note that I will be adding more recipes to the resource page (http://bit.ly/cheerfiles) over the course of the next few months to keep things exciting. You'll also notice that I haven't included any pictures – that's to keep the cost of this book down to a minimum. But if you'd like to see how most of these recipes *should* turn out, visit the website and they should be up in the coming weeks. Finally, if you have any recipe ideas that you'd like to see included on the site, email me: info@thecheerdiet.com (Please be sure to do your homework and include the important numbers such as protein, carb and fat amounts. Finally, don't forget to mention your full name along with your social media links so people can follow you).

Now, let's making something delicious!

Low Carb/Low Cal Meals

Easy Chicken & Rice

This is a recipe I posted on the Instagram account (minus the rice). By the way, you can follow us here: http://instagram.com/thecheerdiet. This recipe is so simple, an ape could manage it. Let's begin:

- 4 large skinless chicken breasts
- Pasta sauce
- ½ tbsp grass-fed butter
- 2 Cups Uncle Ben's instant brown rice
- 1 tbsp crushed red pepper flakes
- 1 tsp cinnamon
- ½ tsp garlic powder
- ½ tsp paprika

In a small bowl, pour in ½ or 1 cup of instant pasta sauce and combine all the spices and butter, then mix into a paste. Place your chicken breasts in the bowl and rub the spice mix all over the chicken. Place chicken on the baking pan, cover with aluminum foil (leave a small gap/opening) and bake at 400°F (200° C) for 50 minutes, then shut off the oven and let the chicken sit for another 10-15 minutes. The internal chicken temp should be at least 165° F (75°C) so make sure you use a meat thermometer to check. This is for your safety.

As for the rice, Uncle Ben's usually comes with instructions on how to make it so follow that, then top with a light amount of salt and pepper. **The recipe produces 4 servings.** Therefore, one meal equals 1 chicken breast with ½ cup of brown rice.

(Nutrition stats per serving)
Protein: 35g
Carbs: 22g
Fats: 13g

Vegetable Omelette

- 3 Large Eggs
- Green Pepper (chopped)
- Tomato (chopped)
- Onion (chopped)
- ½ Tbsp butter

Crack the eggs in a bowl, throw in spices that you like (I use pre-mixed Italian seasoning but just salt and pepper will do just fine) then use a fork to beat until it's runny.

Pre heat non-stick frying pan on medium high, then throw in the butter – wait till the butter melts and becomes bubbly then toss in a handful of each of the vegetables mentioned above (you can use any type of vegetables you like by the way). Cook lightly for about a minute, constantly stirring, then pour in the eggs. Cook the omelette until the top is only very slightly runny, then use a spatula to flip. You know it's cooked perfectly when the omelette is:

A) Not runny
B) Firm enough to be flipped/folded

Once both sides are cooked, fold in half and enjoy! This recipe produces one serving

(Nutrition stats per serving)
Protein: 18g
Carbs: 19g
Fats: 20g

Tuna & Mushroom Omlette

- 2 Large Eggs
- 3 Mushrooms (chopped)
- ½ Can chunk white tuna
- ½ Tbsp butter

Crack the eggs in a bowl, throw in spices that you like (I use pre-mixed Italian seasoning but just salt and pepper will do) then use a fork to beat until it's runny.

Pre heat non-stick frying pan on medium high, then throw in the butter – wait till the butter melts and becomes bubbly then toss in the tuna and mushrooms. Cook lightly until mushrooms are golden, then pour in the eggs. Cook the omelette until the top is only very slightly runny, then use a spatula to flip. You know it's cooked perfectly when the omelette is:

A) Not runny
B) Firm enough to be flipped/folded

Once both sides are cooked, fold in half and enjoy! This recipe produces one serving

(Nutrition stats per serving)
Protein: 28g
Carbs: 5g
Fats: 15g

Coach Sahil's Famous Scrambled Eggs

You won't ever see me boasting about my cooking skills but if there's one thing I can make that can rock anyone's world, its scrambled eggs. Try this recipe – you'll be blown away. Plus, it goes well with steamed vegetables or can be combined with a smoothie since it's already low in calories (yes even in phase one and two).

- 2 Eggs
- 1 Tbsp butter
- Sriracha sauce
- Miss Vickie's Jalapeno Chips (or any kettle cooked chips you like)

Preheat non-stick pan on medium high, then place butter. Wait till butter is bubbly then crack your eggs and throw them into the pan. As soon as the eggs hit the pan, start stirring *constantly*. You don't have to be fast, but keep stirring until your eggs reach the consistently you like. Once done, place scrambled eggs in a bowl – now comes the best bit. Crush about 4-5 chips (find big pieces) until they're basically crumbs. Sprinkle these crumbs over your scrambled eggs then lightly drizzle with sriracha sauce. Enjoy the explosion of pure deliciousness in your mouth. If you can't handle spice, replace sriracha sauce with something milder (but where's the fun in that?). This recipe produces one serving.

(Nutrition stats per serving)
Protein: 12g
Carbs: 4g
Fats: 21g

The Big Bird Meatloaf

- 1 lbs lean ground chicken
- 1 lbs lean ground turkey
- ½ tbsp coconut oil
- ½ cup chicken stock
- 1 and ½ tsp tomato paste
- 1 onion (diced)
- Pinch of garlic powder
- 1 cup bread crumbs
- 1 Egg (beat)
- ¼ cup cheese (parmesan is preferred)
- ¼ cup skim milk
- Salt and pepper

In a pan, combine coconut oil, onion, salt, pepper and garlic powder and cook the onions for about 5 minutes (or until they're a bit see-through). Add in the chicken stock and tomato paste then mix well and let cool.

Combine the ground meats, bread crumbs, egg, skim milk and cheese in a large bowl then mix well. Throw in the onion mixture then mix again. Spread the loaf into a sheet pan, lightly spread any type of sauce you'd like on top. Bake at 400°F (200° C) for about 45 minutes, or until the internal temp reaches 165° F (75°C). Once done, divide the rectangular meatloaf into six even pieces.

(Nutrition stats per serving)
Protein: 42g
Carbs: 16g
Fats: 19g

Beef Kebobs

- 1 pound lean beef cut into one inch cubes
- 2 red bell peppers (cut into 1-2 inch chunks)
- 2 green bell peppers (cut into 1-2 inch chunks)
- 2 cups mushrooms (chopped)
- 1 cucumber (cut into half inch thick slices)
- ½ cup teriyaki sauce
- 1/3 cup honey
- 1 tbsp Sriracha sauce (or any hot sauce you like)
- Pinch of ground ginger powder
- Skewers

Combine the teriyaki sauce, honey, Sriracha sauce, and ginger powder into a bowl and mix. On your skewers, slide on the chunk of beef followed by one piece of each vegetable. The number of skewers you'll get depend on how long they are. Once your kebobs are ready, smear them with our sauce using your hands or a sauce brush.

Preheat grill on medium-high heat for a few minutes and make sure the grate is lightly oiled so nothing sticks. Cook from anywhere to 7-10 minutes till the meat is cooked and the vegetables are tender to your taste.

One serving = ½ the quantities listed, or in other words, if you made 6 skewers, one serving would be 3 skewers.

(Nutrition stats per serving)
Protein: 60g
Carbs: 18g
Fats: 14.5g

Easy Chicken Quinoa

- 1/2 cup Quinoa
- 1 skinless chicken breast, chopped into small slices or cubes
- 3 of your favorite vegetables, chopped into small pieces
- Salt
- Pepper
- Garlic powder
- BBQ sauce
- ½ tbsp coconut oil

Be sure to clean your Quinoa (rinse and wash). Place a pot or sauce pan on stove, and bring about 1 ¼ cups (~330ml) of water to a boil, then add in the Quinoa until all water is absorbed (usually takes around 15 minutes or so). Add in your chopped vegetables along with a pinch of salt, pepper and garlic powder. Or you may use any other spices you like. Stir until vegetables are lightly cooked and everything is evenly mixed then place in a bowl.

To cook the chicken, pre heat pan then throw in the coconut oil. Add all the chicken to pan at once, then season with a pinch of salt and pepper. Stir and cook for 7-8 minutes until chicken is golden brown (also check one of the cubes to make sure the internal temp is 160° F). Once the chicken is just about cooked, throw on some bbq sauce and stir until sauce is evenly applied to every piece. Place chicken on top of Quinoa and enjoy! This recipe makes one serving.

(Nutrition stats per serving)
Protein: 38g
Carbs: 20g
Fats: 14g

Chocolate Banana Oatmeal

- 1/3 cup (30 g) Quaker 1 minute oatmeal
- 1 tbsp Real Maple Syrup
- 1/2 scoop chocolate whey protein powder
- 2/3 cups (160 ml) water
- 1 medium banana, sliced
- Cinnamon powder

In a bowl, place oatmeal, water, maple syrup and protein powder and mix gently for a few minutes. Don't worry if there are clumps for now, just mix it enough so it cooks properly. Place in microwave and cook on high for 60-80 seconds. Mix everything again and you'll notice all clumps disappear easily and you should have a nice creamy, chocolaty oatmeal mix.

Allow a few minutes for the mixture to cool. Now peel and slice the banana to the thickness you like, throw it in and top it off with a pinch of cinnamon powder. Mix everything and enjoy this delicious treat!

(Nutrition stats per serving)
Protein: 17g
Carbs: 47g
Fats: 5g

Meat Rollups

I know, the name sounds terrible but this recipe is actually very simple and super delicious. It literally takes 5 minutes to make.

- 6 Deli meat slices (turkey, chicken, pork or roast beef)
- Spinach
- Kale
- Garlic powder
- Ground pepper
- Chili powder
- Ginger powder

Wash spinach and kale, then cut them into thin, long slices or chunks. You don't have to be perfect, but don't cut them too small - try and make sure their length is about that of your deli meats. Now combine a teaspoon of all the spices in a small cup and mix. Lay down a slice of the deli meat, sprinkle a pinch of the spices on the meat slice (don't go overboard with this), place a bunch of strips of spinach and kale, wrap the meal slice up tightly and eat!

Or, to save it for later, find some baking string to keep the roll ups together. Six meat rollups make one meal.

(Nutrition stats per serving)
Protein: 21g
Carbs: 5g
Fats: 2.5g

Upgraded Celery Sticks

- Celery
- 4 tbsp Nut butter (peanut, almond, cashew or macadamia)
- Raisins

Simply fill the hollow portion of a celery stick with your favorite nut butter until everything is levelled. Place your raisins on top in a line, making sure they're evenly spaced out. Enjoy!

Since celery is so low in calories (and everything else) the portions of this recipe depend solely on the amount of nut butter used. As soon as you've used up 4 tbsp, that equals one meal. You may spread these 4 tbsps through as many celery sticks as you like. So if want to use up an entire tbsp on one celery stick, go for it. Just don't exceed 4 tbsp total, or it becomes more than one meal.

(Nutrition stats per serving)
Protein: 16g
Carbs: 19g
Fats: 32g

Stilton Cheese Salad (recipe from a fan!)

This recipe was generously sent to me by Natalie Byun on Instagram (follow her @byunnana).

- Salad Base Chopped (romaine lettuce, arugula, chard, spinach, cucumber)
- 6 Organic Deli Ham slices
- 1 oz (28g) White Stilton Cheese
- 2 Tbsp Balsamic Vinegar Dressing
- Baguette (Natalie uses 2 slices but to keep carbs low, we shall use 1)

Wash the greens and cucumbers and slice them into desired sizes (quantity of greens depends on size of bowl – fill it up). Slice the ham into small squares. Mix the dressing and greens together. Put the greens + dressing on a plate, and sprinkle the sliced cucumber and ham on top. Crumble some cheese on top, too.

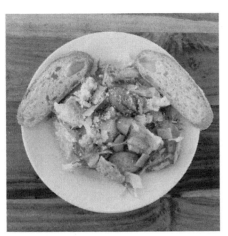

(Nutrition stats per serving)
Protein: 28g
Carbs: 39g
Fat: 15g

Here's a beautiful picture of what it looks like. ©2014 Natalie Byun – image used with permission.

Greek Yogurt Stuffed Strawberries

- 10 fresh strawberries, rinsed & patted dry
- 1 cup of 2% Vanilla Greek Yogurt
- 2 Graham crackers
- 10 fresh Blueberries, rinsed & patted dry

Cut off the strawberry stems, then using a paring knife or melon baller, cut around the inside of the strawberry, hollowing it out slightly and creating a well for the Greek Yogurt. Cut off a small portion of the pointy strawberry tip, so that each strawberry can stand on its own, and place them on a large baking sheet. Use a small spoon and stuff each strawberry with Greek Yogurt, adding a little extra to the top. Stick a blueberry on top of each strawberry. Now to finish it off, crush the graham crackers in a bowl, then sprinkle the crumbs on top of each stuffed strawberry (this step is optional).

Note: Don't make more than 3-4 hours in advance, or your strawberries will become a bit soggy. Any leftover Greek Yogurt can be used as a dip – use the entire cup to complete a meal and hit your protein numbers.

(Nutrition stats per serving)
Protein: 22g
Carbs: 35g
Fat: 5g

Greek Yogurt & Almonds

I'm not even sure you can call this a recipe, but I had to include it because it's so simple – perfect if you're short on time. It literally takes 30 seconds to put together (I'm serious, time yourself and you shall see).

- 1 cup vanilla Greek yogurt (use 0%, 1% or 2% - doesn't matter)
- ½ cup almonds

Put Greek yogurt into a bowl. Throw the almonds on top. Enjoy! This recipe equals one low-carb meal.

(Nutrition stats per serving)
Protein: 37g
Carbs: 22g
Fat: 4.7g

High Carb/High Calorie Meals

Nutella & Banana Sandwich

- 1 Tbsp Nutella
- 2 Slices whole wheat bread
- 1 Medium Banana, Sliced
- 1 Scoop whey protein mixed with 1% milk

Peel and chop banana into slices – thickness depends on personal preference. Slightly toast your bread and spread Nutella on top of one slice followed by sticking the banana slices to it. Now place the other slice of bread on top, and enjoy! To complete this meal, please be sure to eat this sandwich with a whey protein shake (this is reflected in the nutrition information listed below).

(Nutrition stats per serving – with protein shake)
Protein: 41g
Carbs: 45g
Fat: 10g

Home Made Burgers & Salad

- ½ pound lean ground beef (90% or higher)
- Salad Base Chopped (romaine lettuce, arugula, chard, spinach, cucumber)
- Whole wheat burger bun
- Spices: Salt, pepper, cayenne pepper, garlic powder, paprika
- 2 Tbsp Sriracha sauce
- Ketchup
- Olive oil

In a bowl, throw in you your ground beef and a pinch of all the spices plus the Sriracha sauce and a squirt of ketchup. Use your hands to mix it all up until everything is even. Grab a handful of the burger mix and mould into patties (or one SUPER patty). Place on a a tray and toss in the freezer for 10-15 minutes to make them firm. While the patties are hardening, grab a handful of each of the greens, rinse and throw them in a regular sized bowl. *Lightly* top with your favorite dressing and some bread crumbs. Lightly toast your burger bun and keep it ready.

Once the patties (or patty) are slightly hardened, preheat pan on medium-high, put in a tsp of olive oil and cook each side for 2-3 minutes or till internal temp reaches 160°F (71°C). You may top your burger with some tomatoes as a topping if you wish, but nothing more. If you created more than one patty, go ahead have the extra patty topped with your salad. **Do not** exceed one burger bun per meal.

(Nutrition stats per serving)
Protein: 48g
Carbs: 31g
Fat: 20g

Tuna pizza & Chocolate Milk

- 1 can chunk white tuna (in water, not oil)
- BBQ seasoning (or any spice mix you like)
- 1 whole wheat pita bread
- Pasta sauce
- Mozeralla cheese
- Chopped mushrooms and bell pepper
- 1 Cup chocolate milk

Spread pasta sauce over your pita bread, then top with freshly ground black pepper to give it a kick. Evenly spread your chopped mushrooms and bell peppers over the pita and *lightly* top with shredded mozzarella cheese. Preheat pan on medium-high with 1 tsp olive oil, throw in your tuna and sprinkle with bbq seasoning. Cook the tuna for a minute or two while stirring constantly. Now evenly spread the tuna on your pizza and again, top it *lightly* with mozzarella cheese and cook the entire pizza for 12-15 minutes at 375°F depending on your oven. Enjoy with a glass of delicious chocolate milk!

(Nutrition stats per serving – without chocolate milk)
Protein: 43.2g
Carbs: 42g
Fat: 10g

(Nutrition stats per serving – with chocolate milk)
Protein: 51g
Carbs: 69g
Fat: 12.5g

Note: You may substitute the chocolate milk with regular milk or even a protein shake if you like.

Vanilla Spice Blueberry Oatmeal

This is a hearty recipe for champions – one of my favorites to eat about an hour or two before a tough training session. But be warned, eating this on your lazy days is a good way to become plump.

- 1/3 cup (30 g) Quaker 1 minute oatmeal
- 1 scoop vanilla whey protein powder
- ¼ tsp vanilla extract
- 1 tbsp flax seed oil
- 1 tsp raw brown sugar
- ¾ cups (177 ml) water
- 1 Tbsp Peanut Butter
- ½ cup blueberries, rinsed
- ¼ cup raisins
- ¼ cup crushed walnuts
- Spices: cinnamon powder, nutmeg

In a bowl, place oatmeal, water, protein powder, flax oil, brown sugar and mix for a few minutes. Don't worry if there are clumps for now, just mix it enough so it cooks properly. Place in microwave and cook on high for 1.5 minutes. Mix everything again and you should have a nice thick oatmeal mix. Now add in the blueberries, raisins, walnuts, peanut butter, vanilla extract and mix. Sprinkle on nutmeg and cinnamon powder and enjoy!

(Nutrition stats per serving)
Protein: 38.5
Carbs: 54g
Fats: 31g

Steak & Veggie Stir Fry

- 8oz Steak (lean cut, not T-bone)
- Veggies Chopped (carrots, onion, green/red/yellow bell peppers, mushrooms)
- Spices: Garlic powder, paprika, onion powder, cayenne pepper, black pepper, chili powder
- Teriyaki sauce
- Olive oil
- Butter

The amount of veggies you use is up to you – go nuts. Heat olive oil in a pan on high until it just about starts to smoke. Throw in all of your chopped vegetables, and while stirring constantly, throw in a tbsp of teriyaki sauce (or however much you want) along with salt and black pepper. Keep stirring and cooking for about 3-5 minutes or until the onions are browned.

For the steak: Make sure it's at room temperature so that it cooks quickly, and doesn't have a cold center. In a bowl, throw in 2 teaspoons of each of the spices and mix. Now toss your steak in the bowl and make sure that it's evenly covered with the spices. There are many ways to cook a steak, I like mine medium (160° F, 71°C). Pre-heat the pan on high and throw in a tbsp of olive oil. Once the oil starts to smoke, toss in your steak and cook about 2 – 2.5 minutes then flip. As soon as you flip, toss in a small chunk of butter and let the steak cook for another 2 minutes or so. Once cooked, pick up the steak with tongs and squeeze any excess fat into the pan and place on a plate. Sprinkle on any of your left over spices if you'd like. (***Note:*** *an 8oz steak is equal to two portions, so for this meal, you must cut it in half. Use the left over steak for another meal – cook some extra veggies in advance*)

(Nutrition stats per serving – half the steak plus vegetables)
Protein: 30g
Carbs: 25g
Fats: 18g

Chicken Nuggets & Squash

- 3 skinless chicken breasts
- 1 Cup seasoned bread crumbs
- ½ cup finely grated cheese (any type you like)
- 1 tsp dried thyme, crushed as finely as possible
- 1 tsp ground black pepper
- 1 tsp garlic powder
- 1 tsp chili powder
- 1 tbsp dried basil, crushed
- ½ cup melted butter
- 1 cup butternut squash

In a bowl, mix together all of the ingredients except the butter, squash and chicken. Chop the chicken breasts into 1 inch sized cubes (or however big you want your nuggets to be). Have a separate bowl with the melted butter in it, ready to go. Now dip the chicken cubes in the melted butter first, then toss in the breadcrumb mixture and coat evenly. Place the chicken piece on a lightly greased cookie sheet or baking pan. Once all the chicken nuggets are ready to go, preheat over at 400° F (205° C) and cook for about 20 minutes until the nuggets are golden brown. Double check that the internal temperature of the nuggets is at least 165° F (75°C). Microwave your squash for a minute so that it's easier to cut, now chop it into small cubes and toss in a bowl. Drizzle some of your leftover butter over the squash and mix well until evenly coated (don't add too much). Season with any of the spices you like, or use any leftover breadcrumb mix. Place the seasoned squash on a baking sheet, cover with foil and bake at 400° F (205° C) for 15 minutes, then flip the pieces and cook for another 15 minutes. *(Note: the chicken nuggets makes 3 servings, so if you made 30 nuggets, use only 10 with your 1 cup of squash)*

(Nutrition stats per serving – 1/3 of the nuggets with squash)
Protein: 35g
Carbs: 45g
Fats: 38g

Spicy Beef Chilli

- 1 pound lean ground beef
- 1 Onion, chopped and diced
- 1 green bell pepper, chopped and diced
- Garlic (1 clove, minced)
- 1 Can of beans (black or kidney)
- ½ chipotle pepper, chopped (omit if you don't like spicy)
- 1 can crushed tomatoes
- 1 Can beef broth (low sodium if possible)
- Premade chili seasoning mix

In a pan, pre heat on medium high and add in 1 tsp olive oil. Now add in ground beef and cook for a few minutes until lightly browned. Add in the diced onion, garlic, and chipotle pepper and cook for another 3-5 minutes (do not overcook the beef). Now throw the beef/veggie mix into a large pot and add in the rest of the ingredients and bring to a boil while stirring. Now reduce heat to medium and cook for 20-30 min until the chili reaches your desired level of thickness. If it becomes too thick, you may always add water. (**Note:** The amount of chili seasoning to use depends on your taste, start with 1.5 tbsp and do a taste test as it cooks. Add more if you like. One meal serving equals 1.5 cups of the chilli)

(Nutrition stats per serving)
Protein: 45g
Carbs: 61g
Fats: 37g

Fruit & Nut Energy Bars

- 1 cup mixed nuts (pick any three you like. Examples: almonds, walnuts, peanuts, macadamia etc.)
- 1 cup mixed dried fruit (pick a few you like. Examples: Apricots, Figs, Pineapple, Mango, Raisins, Papaya, Black Currant, Plum etc.)
- 1 cup Medjool seedless dates
- Food processor, wax paper, baking

Throw the nuts, dried fruit, and dates in a food processor and start with a few pulses to break it all up. If things start to clump, you will have to separate it. Keep processing until everything is turned into crumb-sized pieces. Scrape the edges of the container and the blade to make sure nothing is sticking. Continue processing until the ingredients clump/bind together and gather into a ball (will take anywhere from 5-10 minutes). Lay a piece of plastic wrap or wax paper on your baking sheet, place your big clump of material and chill in the freezer for 5-10 minutes. Now press the dough until it forms a thick square, roughly 8" x 8" in size. Wrap it up and chill either overnight in the fridge or for 15 minutes in the freezer. Once you've chilled it, transfer the dough on to a cutting board and cut into 8 large bars. In the fridge, these bars can last for several weeks or a couple months in the freezer. I prefer eating them chilled, but at room temperature they're a bit softer and still delicious.

One meal is equal to 2 of these bars. They make for an excellent pre-workout meal before a training session. Be sure to drink lots of water.

(Nutrition stats – per 2 bars)
Protein: 8.2g
Carbs: 84.5g
Fats: 18g

Smoothie Recipes

While the food recipes mentioned earlier are absolutely delicious, I think your taste buds are in for a real treat when you try the smoothies I have lined up for you. Holly and I spent almost an entire day trying out different combinations (and making a huge mess in the kitchen), until we found ones that are nutritious and delicious. We hope you enjoy drinking these smoothies as much as we enjoyed coming up with them.

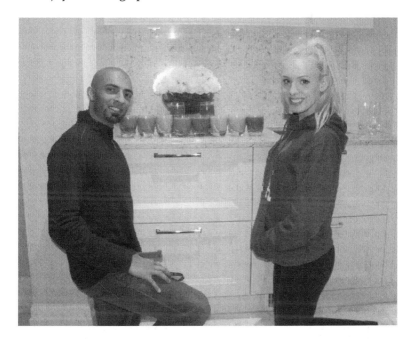

Also, I wanted to take a second to thank a young lady named Maddie Stark for being an invaluable assistant during the smoothie testing phase. If it wasn't for her meticulous note taking skills, this section wouldn't exist, so be sure to follow her on IG and say something nice: @maddie__stark (that's a double underscore)

Getting Started

Before you blitz up a bunch of fruits and veggies into something drinkable, there is one key item which you'll need to get your hands on - a **powerful** blender. Initially we tried using the MagicBullet™ which was ok, but it had a habit of leaving behind chunks every once in a while. And nobody likes chunks. However, when the recipes were re-tested with a more powerful blender (Vitamix™) the difference was night and day. Combinations that I thought needed changing magically started to work, just because they were blended together better.

Here's a quick test – if you have to ask, "Will this blend?" after fill up a blender container with the ingredients, then you probably need to invest in a machine that can pulverize anything that stands in its way. Based on what I've seen Blendtec™ blenders do (turn an iPhone into fine pixie dust) I'm sure a few berries and ice cubes won't pose much of a threat, so maybe consider getting one of those.

Vitamix™ info: http://thecheerdiet.com/links/vitamix
Blendtec™ info: http://thecheerdiet.com/links/blendtec

Speaking of consistency, it should be noted that every smoothie recipe was made with ice and water. How much of each? That depends on your taste – if you like your smoothies so thick that you go blue in the face trying to suck it up through a straw, use two handfuls of ice and little bit of water. But if you're normal (like me), use more water to keep it drinkable. Next, to turn any of these recipes into a post-workout smoothie, just add one scoop of whey protein powder (favored or unflavored, it doesn't matter). By themselves, these smoothies consist purely of carbohydrates, designed to be consumed within 40-60 minutes of your training session to give you the fuel you need. But muscles that have been worked to their limits need more than carbs to recover (as you very well know by now), and whey protein is an excellent choice.

As for prep, each ingredient was washed, peeled if necessary, and chopped into regular sized chunks so that we could use a handful. Thus, "a handful" became our standard unit of measure (I know, so scientific right?). You might be wondering if frozen ingredients are an option, and the answer is absolutely. But if you have the time, try using fresh organic produce since you can really taste the difference.

Also remember that nothing is written in stone - if there is an ingredient that you really like, feel free to throw in a little extra. And this brings us to the most important point when it comes to consuming the smoothies – portion size. When following the protocols of the diet, each smoothie serving is to be kept **strictly at 350ml (or 1.5 cups).** If you end up making any extra, share with your friends, or your coaches (a very good idea), or refrigerate for later use. The pictures of what these smoothies look like can be found on the resource page (along with some bonus, behind the scene shots which are quite hilarious).

Now let's make some smoothies!

Smoothie #1
- watermelon
- kale
- apple
- blueberries
- banana
- splash of orange juice
- 2 tbsp yogurt

Smoothie #2
- strawberries
- spinach
- watermelon
- small piece of ginger, grated
- pear
- splash of orange juice

Smoothie #3
- mango
- half a banana
- raspberries
- watermelon
- splash of peach juice
- 2 tbsp vanilla yogurt

Smoothie #4
- watermelon
- blackberries
- carrots
- pear
- apple
- splash of orange & peach juice

Smoothie #5
- spinach
- small piece of ginger, grated
- 1 tsp lemon juice
- banana (whole)
- kale
- splash of orange & peach juice
- strawberries
- pear
- raspberries
- mango

Smoothie #6 (Holly's Creation)
- mango
- splash of peach juice
- strawberries
- apple
- banana (half)
- blueberries
- 1 tbsp honey

Smoothie #7 (Maddie's Creation)
- strawberries
- mango
- raspberries
- carrots
- splash of peach juice
- pear
- honey

Smoothie #8
- blueberries
- strawberries
- blackberries
- raspberries
- spinach
- splash of tart cherry juice
- honey

Smoothie #9
- carrots
- cilantro (little bit)
- kale
- spinach
- small piece of ginger, grated
- splash of lemon & orange juice
- oranges

Smoothie #10
- blueberries
- pear
- banana
- apple
- splash of tart cherry & peach juice
- optional (2 tbsp vanilla yogurt)

Chapter 7: Training While On The Cheer Diet

The three phases of this diet were designed based on the assumption that you're a serious all-star cheerleader who trains a minimum of 3 times per week (ideally 4).

But what if you're not a cheerleader? Can you still follow the diet?

Of course! I want to make sure that *any* female athlete who picks up my book has a chance to reap its benefits, regardless of her chosen sport or activity. However, we all know that training intensity differs from one sport to the next, so to level the playing field and make sure you're not overfeeding yourself, I'm going to show you a tool I use called RPE. Think of it as your training compass – it'll always help point you in the right direction.

Understanding RPE (Rate of Perceived Exertion)

It may sound like a bunch of fancy words strung together, but in plain English RPE just means *"how hard do you think you worked, on a scale of 1-10?"*

Let me give you a few examples: If someone asked me to do a round off back handspring, my RPE would be about 4/10 because this is a skill I've been doing for a long time. But ask a level 2 athlete that just learnt this pass, and their RPE is probably a 9/10.

Or let's say I deadlifted 400lbs at the gym today; my RPE would be 9.8/10 since the max I've ever done is 405. However, ask Benedikt Magnusson to pull the same amount of weight, and his RPE will most likely be 3/10 since his max is over 1000lbs!

I think you get the idea – only *you* can really assess your RPE. So how does this relate to the diet?

Simple, if your RPE is under 7/10 for a training session then either you need to supplement it with an extra workout, or write it off as a rest day. A perfect example is choreography day – sure you're in the gym and working, but you're not really pushing yourself like you are at tumbling or stunting practice.

So either you write off your choreography session as a rest day, or spend a good chunk of time afterwards doing some serious conditioning. If you need a good conditioning program, Holly and I have put together a great video for you right here:

http://youtu.be/_GMg7ODULZg

For each exercise that you see in the video, start a timer for 60 seconds and do as many clean repetitions as possible. Assuming you do all of the exercises and push yourself, the workout should take you about 20 minutes and produce an RPE of about 7 or 8.

The reason I like using RPE as a tool is that it forces you to be honest with yourself. You can lie to your coaches, parents and friends by saying something like, *"OMG just did a conditioning program that felt like an RPE of 9/10!"* Then use it as an excuse to eat some high carb meals, but a month down the road your lack of results will be clearly visible. You are not immune to the laws of Thermodynamics.

Here are two examples of what an ideal week would look like for a cheerleader following the diet:

Example 1 – Training 3x a week

Mon	Tue	Wed	Thurs	Fri	Sat	Sun
Cheer	Rest	Cheer	Rest	Rest	Tumbling	Rest
RPE: 7		RPE: 7			RPE: 8	

Example 2 – Training 4x a week

Mon	Tue	Wed	Thurs	Fri	Sat	Sun
Cheer	Rest	Cheer	Rest	Tumbling	Rest	Cheer
RPE: 7		RPE: 7		RPE: 9		RPE: 8

Chapter 8: Frequently Asked Questions

While this book is a new release, below are some of the questions that clients (including athletes) usually ask me when I create diet plans for them, and most can be applied to *The Cheer Diet* as well. After so many years, I've found that nutrition questions are usually universal and should you have any, they're most likely covered in this section.

However, if I happened to miss, feel free to email me here: info@thecheerdiet.com. Onwards we go...

Q: "Am I allowed to have some junk food on TCD? I know being healthy is important but I also want to live, enjoy life and not be a social outcast!"

Of course, remember that after phase one you get a cheat day where you can have whatever you want, and once you're in phase three, you can not only have some HG carbs before your training session, but you get one cheat day every 2 weeks, which is about **24 cheat days per year.** That's almost a month's worth of days where you can enjoy hanging with your girls, and eating whatever you want.

But remember that to ensure long-term success, cultivating a habit is very important. So for the first two phases, you will definitely be stressing that willpower muscle of yours. DO NOT be afraid of becoming *that* friend who has become "the health nut."

If your friends or family members are teasing you or making off-hand remarks, just know that it's usually out of jealousy or mis-understanding of your goals. Because let's face it, if the people you hang out with *truly* cared about you, and knew how important cheer is to you, they wouldn't be giving you a hard time, would they?

Didn't think so. So *make them* understand that when you politely refuse their extra food servings, it's not to be insulting. It just isn't in alignment with your goals at the moment. If they still don't get it, just move on with your life or find better friends. Trust me, life is too short to hang around people that just want to bring you down.

Q: "I've gotten used to preparing my meals and making the recipes but what do I do when I'm going to a restaurant for things like team dinners and special occasions?"

This situation is actually very easy to handle. First of all, if you've gotten used to cooking the recipes, then you probably have a good idea of the amount of protein and carbs that are in each meal. You also know when to eat meals with higher carbs and when not to. Based on these factors, you can easily pick menu items that closely resemble the recipes in this book.

So for example, if you're going out for a team dinner after training, you know that taking in protein and good quality carbs is important. And that avoiding simple sugars (such as from soda or cake) is not a great idea. So what would you order?

Well, how about a chicken salad? Or whole wheat pasta with meat balls? Or brown rice and a juicy steak? All of these would make a great post-workout meal. As for rest days, how about a burger? But tell the waiter that you'd like to ditch the top half of the bun and pile on some more veggies instead. You can easily enjoy this type of burger with a fork and knife and it's one of my personal favourite options.

As you can see, it's not rocket science:

1. Figure out the timing (do I eat like it's a rest day, pre training or post training?)
2. Are there any options that closely resemble the recipes I cook at home? If so, that's what I should order.
3. If not, can I make any modifications that make sense?

That's it – a simple three step process. In fact, it can be a two-step process if the restaurant you're visiting has lots of options to choose from. And please, for the love of god, don't over-think this stuff or get stressed out by aiming for perfection.

The point of going out is to socialize and have fun, so just try your best – I promise your diet won't get screwed up. Good enough, is good enough.

Q: "I started phase 2 last week and loving the results, but I feel slightly tired on my rest days, is this normal and is there anything I can do?"

If you've never paid attention to the way you eat based on your body's needs before then yes, it's absolutely normal. Remember that while your body does store excess calories as fat, it also get used to a higher fuel intake – especially if you've been doing this for years.

This habit will not go away immediately, which is why phase 1 exists. To fully adapt, it might take another week, or it could take all 60 days. It all depends on how many years you've been neglecting your diet. So just be patient, but in the mean time you can also rely on the help of coffee to keep your mental state alert.

Now remember, you shouldn't have more than two cups in a day, and it has to be actual coffee; black if possible or with a splash of cream and just a hint of sugar for taste. Green tea would be preferable. The natural caffeine from these beverages can give you a boost when you need it – such as powering through homework. Finally, don't forget to ensure that you're taking in adequate fats on your rest days. If you forget to take your fish oils in the morning and aren't cooking the recipes exactly as they're designed, that might be why you're feeling more tried than usual.

Q: "I don't mind the recipes but I want to experiment with others and add some more variety to the diet. Is there any way that I can add my own?"

Absolutely – but only once you're on phase 3. If you'll notice, the macronutrient breakdown of each recipe is listed, which means that you can totally come up with your own or look up other recipes that you want to try – just be sure to modify them to match the numbers listed in the book.

As an example, a can of tuna and a skinless chicken breast have around the same amount of protein (27-30 grams) so instead of making chicken salad, you can find a recipe for tuna salad and replace the veggies with ones you like.

The variations and combinations that you can come up with are basically endless, and I definitely encourage you to play around and have fun with it. At the end of the day, you're more likely to stick with a diet when it's completely customized to you.

Q: "Help! I missed the pre-training window because of XYZ reasons, and now I have practice in 20 minutes! Is there anything I can do? I don't want to throw up food, but on the other hand, don't want to feel hungry and tired either!"

First I need to shake my finger at you and reinforce the fact that if there's one part of *The Cheer Diet* where you need to be the most diligent, it's the pre-workout eating window. It is vital that you have lots of energy during practices because it can make the difference between landing a tumbling pass, or busting it. Or catching your flyer on time, versus dropping her. A mentally focused and energized athlete is not only an asset to a team in terms of performance, but also safety.

With that said, the best thing I recommend in such a small timeframe is a small cup of coffee with a piece of low-fibre fruit. A handful of grapes paired with coffee is absolutely perfect for those last minute situations. Also, don't forget to take a can of coconut water with you to drink as you start to sweat.

Why low fibre? Because fibre slows the absorption of nutrients, which is great most of the time, but with practice coming up so quickly, that's the last thing we want. Other fruits you can have at this short of a notice are: watermelon, cantaloupe, pineapple, banana (small ones only).

Another option is simply a glass of chocolate milk (250ml). While the coffee-plus-fruit option is awesome, there's not much protein in there. Also, the great thing about chocolate milk is that it is available nearly everywhere, so it's virtually impossible that you *won't* be able to get your hands on it.

Finally, if your parents are the ones that drop you off to practice, you can create a simple "emergency kit" and leave it in their car. I say kit, but really all you're going to do is throw in a scoop of protein powder into a shaker cup, and keep it stored in a cool dry spot, such as the trunk. Then when the time comes, just grab the cup, throw in some water, shake it and drink up!

Q: "Coach, I train about 6 days per week and I swear my RPE for each of those days is at least a 7, should I still follow the first two phases, and also, when I get to phase 3, should I only take one rest day?"

This is a great question. The answer to the first part is yes – regardless of how much you train, you need to follow the first two phases. Now when you get to phase 3 and your volume of training is this high, then you need to take a moment and think about which of your six training sessions is the least tiring. I promise you can find one.

For this diet to work and produce results, you need to eat the rest day meal plan for a minimum of two days out of the week (and a maximum of four). What this will do is put your body is in a very small caloric deficit – thus guaranteeing that you burn fat as fuel, and keep yourself insulin sensitive (this is a good thing). Eating high carb/high calorie for six days is not something I recommend.

My Outro

I wanted to thank you again for supporting my work. If you found this book informative and enjoyable, it would mean the world if you took a few seconds to Tweet, Facebook, or Instagram'ed about it to spread the word. A review on Amazon would also go a long way.

Being an independent author isn't easy – there are no early book advances, no marketing departments with massive budgets to promote the work, and no publicist with a laundry list of connections to help give this project a jump start. It's just me, my laptop and the desire to write about ideas that will help others. So every social media mention, regardless of how many followers you have, is an act I'm thankful for.

On the flipside, being indie does have its perks; for one, there is no boss, so I get to call *all* the shots. Second, there is no set deadline to hit except those I make for myself. Finally, I get to update this book as often as I'd like, which means I get to treat it like an app.

What you hold in your hand is version 1.0, so it's very likely that you may have come across little quirks or "bugs" along the way (if so, please email me: info@thecheerdiet.com). But it also means that I will release updated editions in the future, and as an early adopter, you'll get access to those updates **for free** (they'll be available as PDF downloads). Heck, I may even release an *actual* app if I have the time and resources to do so.

Finally, if there's a slight chance that this book has peaked your interest in the area of nutrition, biology or anything else that involves helping people become the best they can be, then maybe I can help guide your way. You see, one common question I get asked by my peers and fellow coaches in the tumbling/cheer world is, *"where the heck did you learn all this nutrition stuff?"* and my answer is, *"Through endless experimentation and from people much smarter than myself."* Or in other words, I stand on the shoulders of giants.

If you go to the book resource page (http://bit.ly/cheerfiles - password is **tcd2015**), you'll find a list of people who I've personally learnt a lot from. They're not only intellectually brilliant, but they've all helped real athletes achieve real results. They are the experts whom other experts look up to, so I highly recommend checking out their work. You won't be disappointed.

Train hard, eat well and stay fierce.

Share on Twitter

Share on Facebook

Coach Sahil M.
Certified Level 2 Gymnastics Coach
Former National Champion
Nutritional Consultant
Founder of Addicted To Tumbling

Table Of Contents

References For Chapter 1

1. http://www.webmd.com/diet/healthy-kitchen-11/truth-about-gluten
2. http://www.packagedfacts.com/Gluten-Free-Foods-7144767/
3. http://www.ncbi.nlm.nih.gov/pubmed/23648697
4. http://news.nationalpost.com/2012/11/24/canadas-organic-food-certification-system-little-more-than-an-extortion-racket-report-says/
5. http://ajcn.nutrition.org/content/early/2010/01/13/ajcn.2009.277 25.abstract
6. http://circ.ahajournals.org/content/111/5/e89.full
7. http://www.ncbi.nlm.nih.gov/pubmed/1386252
8. http://www.ncbi.nlm.nih.gov/pubmed/19943985
9. http://www.ncbi.nlm.nih.gov/pubmed/9155494
10. http://www.cnn.com/2010/HEALTH/11/08/twinkie.diet.professor
11. http://www.tampabay.com/features/fitness/life-of-pie-losing-weight-by-eating-nothing-but-pizza/1029472
12. http://www.ncbi.nlm.nih.gov/pubmed/20339363
13. http://www.ncbi.nlm.nih.gov/pubmed/3661473
14. http://www.ncbi.nlm.nih.gov/pubmed/10837292
15. http://www.medicalnewstoday.com/articles/134385.php
16. http://www.ncbi.nlm.nih.gov/pubmed/21787904
17. http://www.marathonandbeyond.com/choices/emmett.htm
18. http://www.ncbi.nlm.nih.gov/pubmed/21330616
19. *Sweet Misery, A Poisoned World*
20. *http://examine.com/faq/is-diet-soda-bad-for-you.html*

References For Chapter 2

1. http://www.telegraph.co.uk/health/healthnews/5857845/It-takes-66-days-to-form-a-habit.html
2. http://www.ncbi.nlm.nih.gov/pubmed/9599441
3. *Is Willpower A Limited Resource?*
4. http://www.ncbi.nlm.nih.gov/pubmed/10748642
5. *The Power Of Habit – Charles Duhigg*

References For Chapter 3

1. http://www.ncbi.nlm.nih.gov/pubmed/15282028
2. http://www.ncbi.nlm.nih.gov/pubmed/19394978
3. http://www.ncbi.nlm.nih.gov/pubmed/12904638
4. http://www.ncbi.nlm.nih.gov/pubmed/9040548
5. http://www.ncbi.nlm.nih.gov/pubmed/20164290
6. http://www.ncbi.nlm.nih.gov/pubmed/20511059
7. http://www.ncbi.nlm.nih.gov/pubmed/19451765
8. http://www.ncbi.nlm.nih.gov/pubmed/22087615
9. http://www.ncbi.nlm.nih.gov/pubmed/17055120
10. Jaffe R MD. "How to Know if You are Magnesium Deficient: 75% of Americans Are" (transcript), 06/16/05, www.innovativehealing.com
11. http://www.ncbi.nlm.nih.gov/pubmed/20352370
12. http://www.ncbi.nlm.nih.gov/pubmed/1619184
13. http://www.ncbi.nlm.nih.gov/pubmed/12490960
14. http://www.ncbi.nlm.nih.gov/pubmed/12490959
15. http://www.ncbi.nlm.nih.gov/pubmed/19594223
16. http://www.ncbi.nlm.nih.gov/pubmed/21907450
17. http://www.sciencedirect.com/science/article/pii/S0006899306027144
18. http://www.sciencedirect.com/science/article/pii/S0166432812006997
19. http://www.ncbi.nlm.nih.gov/pubmed/18845707
20. http://www.besthealthmag.ca/eat-well/healthy-eating/6-reasons-to-eat-more-beans-and-lentils
21. http://news.yahoo.com/nycs-bloomberg-led-way-trans-fats-ban-071436988--finance.html
22. http://www.nytimes.com/2013/11/12/opinion/an-overdue-ban-on-trans-fats.html?_r=0
23. http://www.ncbi.nlm.nih.gov/pubmed/12056182

References For Chapter 5

1. http://www.reuters.com/article/2014/04/30/france-happiness-idUSL6N0NM41D20140430
2. http://www.ncbi.nlm.nih.gov/pubmed/21470061
3. http://www.ncbi.nlm.nih.gov/pubmed/9731851
4. http://www.ncbi.nlm.nih.gov/pubmed/11890637

Don't forget to visit www.TheCheerDiet.com for future articles and updates!

If you purchased the digital PDF edition of *The Cheer Diet*, know that an audiobook is in the works and is scheduled for release during the summer of 2015 and you'll get 100% FREE access. For those who've purchased the paperback edition, the audiobook will be available at a steep discount.

Made in the USA
Lexington, KY
20 June 2016